10-MINUTE
PILATES
WITH THE BALL

Lesley Ackland

10-MINUTE
PILATES
WITH THE BALL

Simple routines for a strong, toned body

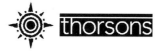

Thorsons
An Imprint of HarperCollins*Publishers*
77–85 Fulham Palace Road,
Hammersmith,
London W6 8JB

The website address is: www.thorsonselement.com

thorsons™

and *Thorsons* are registered trademarks
of HarperCollins*Publishers* Ltd

Published by Thorsons 2003

10 9 8 7 6 5 4 3 2 1

A catalogue record for this book is
available from the British Library

ISBN 0 00 716600 1

Printed and bound in Great Britain by
Martins the Printers Ltd, Berwick upon Tweed

Contents

Acknowledgements

10-Minute Pilates with the Ball would not have been possible without the support and involvement of Nick Ringham for helping with the photo shoots, Julia Daly for the pregnancy case study and photos, Jane Ireland for writing about physiotherapy, Paul Windle and his staff, Carolyn Hunter and, not least, Nupu Press and Malu Halasa.

For further information on the Body Maintenance Studio, send a stamped addressed envelope to:

Body Maintenance Studio
Second Floor
Pineapple
7 Langley Street
London WC2H 9JA

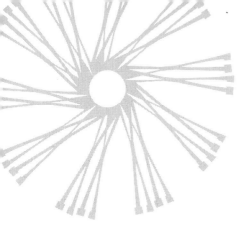

Introduction

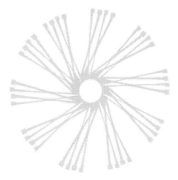

10-Minute Pilates with the Ball is based on my Body Maintenance Technique, a Pilates-based programme which focuses on equal amounts of strengthening and stretching exercises to give you a correct, posturally-aligned body.

THE PHYSIO BALL

Physio Balls are an important tool in my Body Maintenance studio at Pineapple in London's Covent Garden. Currently available in sport shops, Physio Balls are a very simple exercise accessory that can be used almost anywhere – at the studio or at home, even in the office. They don't require a lot of space or time to blow them up; they're not a complicated piece of equipment.

Physio Balls have been a part of Body Maintenance for the last 10 years. When I first introduced them, they weren't widely known. Initially I started using them in my Pilates-based technique because I had learned of their use in advanced physiotherapy therapy taking place in German clinics.

A serious remedial tool, Physio Balls are especially important for patients recovering from surgery, particularly those recovering from spinal surgery (laminectomies). They have also been used at the New York City Ballet and, since then, have been successfully incorporated into most gyms and exercise regimes, where they have proved to be extremely useful.

In the Body Maintenance studio I have devised simple exercises for people recovering from spinal surgery. They are also fantastic for shoulder and spine problems, particularly scoliosis in the upper back. Amazingly, most of my clients now do at least 25 to 30 per cent of their 90-minute programme with a Physio Ball.

From the point of view of strengthening, stabilizing and mobilizing your joints and muscles, Physio Balls are essential. However, it is worth remembering that for people with a serious problem or injury, the use of a Physio Ball must be undertaken only under the guidance of a qualified physiotherapist.

The exercises in this book are not, however, remedial exercises. They are ordinary exercises that have been designed to offer you a varied and challenging programme. The standing and balancing exercises, some of which have been published in my previous books, can be used with or without a Physio Ball – although one of the many pluses of working on a ball is that the exercises are not done standing, so the correct posture can be more easily be achieved.

10-Minute Pilates with the Ball is an exercise routine that is rigorous, but one that does not place undue weight or pressure on the joints. These exercises allow you to focus more on correct posture and correct alignment, without having to worry about gravity in the way that you do when you are standing.

PILATES AND PREGNANCY

In the Body Maintenance studio, working with Physio Balls has been particularly useful for my pregnant clients. The Body Maintenance studio specializes in post- and antenatal work, and we teach pregnant clients right up until a week or two before birth; we also see them anywhere from six weeks after giving birth. A section of this book has been specifically devoted to the weekly exercise programme performed by 10 to 15 of my clients a week in the Body Maintenance studio. You can be confident that they have been tried and tested successfully for a number of years by many women before and after they give birth, week in and week out – some even after their third or fourth child, or after having given birth to twins.

A SHORT HISTORY OF PILATES

Pilates was originally devised by Joseph Pilates, born a sickly child in Germany. His system of gentle physical exercise helped him overcome tuberculosis and go on to become a professional gymnast and athlete.

Interned in Britain during the First World War, he developed his regime for injured soldiers, incorporating pulleys and springs attached to hospital beds, to prevent muscle wastage, maintain strength and increase stamina. Later in Germany, the dancer and choreographer Rudolph von Laban used Pilates' warm-up and stretching techniques for his own dance troupe.

In the 1920s, Pilates moved to the US and opened a clinic in New York City. It soon became a favourite of the dancers and choreographers Martha Graham and George Balanchine, who brought in members of the New York City Ballet. A popular therapy for dancers wanting to work around their injuries, the low-impact exercise system also had early devotees in Hollywood stars like Katharine Hepburn and Lauren Bacall. In recent years, with the lean, youthful look in vogue, Pilates has been picked up by modern celebrities like Madonna and Uma Thurman.

A SHORT HISTORY OF BODY MAINTENANCE

At the time Pilates was created, society was on the whole more active. Many of today's common injuries are a result of our modern lifestyles. Sitting hunched over our desks and having to engage in repetitive movements on computer keyboards, for example, contradict the physiological needs of the human body and create an imbalance. To address these debilitating afflictions of contemporary stress, I knew I had to expand and enhance the basic principles of Pilates.

I began developing Body Maintenance in 1980, initially studying with Alan Herdman, who first brought Pilates to the UK. While continuing my Pilates studies during frequent trips to New York City, I became aware of the extensive research being carried out on the human body. I began looking at the way physiotherapists were working, particularly at the New York City Ballet, with Physio Balls and Dynabands.

Building on a Pilates foundation, I began to incorporate methods from a wide variety of sources, including Alexander Technique, Feldenkrais and even osteopathy, as well as remedial massage and injury clinics. Integrating nutrition and mental improvement with controlled exercise, I created my unique system of bodywork which I call Body Maintenance.

Over the past 15 years in my own studio, I have worked successfully with people who have suffered from a variety of modern infirmities: RSI (carpal tunnel syndrome), chronic back pain (some of which stems from spinal surgery), HIV-related problems, aerobic sprains, extreme obesity, even low self-esteem.

Body Maintenance differs from other forms of exercise because it initially focuses on posture. Good posture is vital in realigning the body, which can have you looking and feeling taller, slimmer and more well toned. Body Maintenance doesn't build bulk, but strengthens weak muscles and stretches out tight ones. You can concentrate on one part of the body without straining another.

Body Maintenance recognizes that exercise is truly effective when you synchronize thought and action. Mentally focusing on the muscle you are using in each exercise is essential. This mind–body technique is the main principle of Body Maintenance. In order to create a fit and healthy body, you need to integrate the mental, physical and spiritual spheres.

Many people, particularly women, do not have a positive body self-image. Using *10-Minute Pilates with the Ball* can help you achieve the body you want and are comfortable with, not the body you think you 'should' have. All too often we are held hostage to images we see in glossy magazines, and imagine they are preferable to the body we've got. I find this unrealistic, even dangerous. We should acknowledge and appreciate our own bodies and work with what we are given. We do have the ability to transform ourselves, to reduce our self-imposed limitations and tap into our potential – using my Body Maintenance techniques in a daily routine will stretch both your body and your mind.

CORE STABILITY

One reason why Physio Balls are an essential tool in Body Maintenance is that exercising with them increases core stability. This is the utilization of the abdominals and the muscles in the spine to create postural integrity that will give you the posture and balance of someone who is much younger and more confident. Better posture and balance helps you to exude vitality and youthfulness.

On the unstable surface of a Physio Ball, the body works harder to achieve the internal stability you would normally get from doing basic abdominal exercises. When my older, more mature clients work on a ball, they unconsciously employ the many muscle groups that we normally don't use to support the body. I believe that the exercises in Body Maintenance really do reverse the effects of gravity and ageing.

Physio Balls also strengthen your 'proprioceptive awareness' – a popular concept in dance and bodywork. This is the unconscious link between mind and body, the physiological connection between the brain and the body. For example, if your proprioceptive awareness is developed and you slip on the street, you're more likely to regain your balance than to lose it. Tripping or falling happen because the lack of co-ordination between your mind and body has increased your chances of losing your balance. The Body Maintenance system of controlled, focused exercise works on strengthening your proprioceptive awareness. Without thought or analysis, the body corrects itself to avoid any mishap or misstep.

The use of Physio Balls in my Pilates-based studio or with a good personal trainer will greatly enhance a return to general fitness and agility.

The Mind–Body Connection

1

Mindful Exercise

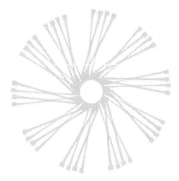

The very essence of Body Maintenance is to harness your thinking to bring about positive changes in your body. By concentrating on a limited number of slow repetitions, you direct your energy towards what you want to achieve. You allow your mind to exert a greater influence over your body. Positive thoughts bring about positive changes.

It is necessary to complement each physical exercise with a mental focus. By practising creative visualization regularly, you gradually develop the intellectual and emotional ability to internalize the physical changes you wish to make. Once you do this, the external changes will start to appear.

Body Maintenance is based on lengthening and stretching the body to its full potential. This eventually creates a longer, leaner shape, increased flexibility and a suppleness that promotes greater ease of movement. These exercises concentrate on strengthening weak muscles and stretching those that are tight and constricted. What you really want is a body in which strength and flexibility complement each other. It is possible to re-structure yourself totally.

This is not, however, just a matter of getting your body to make the right moves. An integral part of Body Maintenance is the way you *perceive* each exercise.

This is where attitude and creative imagery come in. Every time you work through a sequence of movements, it is essential that you envision what it is you want to achieve. Having a mental picture in your mind helps your body to respond in the right way. This not only makes the whole process more stimulating, but also makes the effect of each exercise much more powerful.

Initially it may take a while to understand fully the mechanisms involved. I always tell a new client to expect to do only about 30 percent of what he or she will eventually be capable of doing. Concentrating on the moment will make it possible to remember more each time you practise. It takes about 10 sessions to really comprehend this technique.

Body Maintenance is one of the few forms of exercise that gets progressively more difficult, but the results are worth it. In time you will look taller, slimmer and more toned.

MIND OVER MATTER

Research shows that the mind can induce positive physiological effects on the body, both internal and external. You may notice that when you're in a good mood you automatically seem to look better and feel healthier as well. Scientists ascribe this phenomenon to the activity of billions of nerve cells in our brain which transmit chemical messages to the rest of the body. Our thoughts and emotions play a vital role in influencing this intercellular communication.

Think for a moment about how unpleasant you feel when you're stressed. Your body produces an excess of stress chemicals, like adrenaline and cortisol, which causes your whole system to speed up. Your heart beats faster, your blood pressure goes up, your breathing becomes rapid and shallow. This response is necessary to motivate you in a crisis. But in our day-to-day lives, large doses of this reaction can be extremely harmful and lead to symptoms such as dizziness, profuse sweating, shaking, insomnia and migraines. Tight, tense muscles make your body shrink, constricting the flow of energy throughout the body. This eventually results in a weak, misshapen musculature.

Positive feelings of calm and contentment have a far more beneficial effect. The release of health-enhancing feel-good chemicals, like endorphins and serotonin, are vital for well-being. You breathe more easily and deeply, your heart rate is slower and your blood pressure lowers. This sense of serenity has an overall positive effect on your general bearing and posture.

CREATIVE VISUALIZATION

How you picture yourself is reflected in your body language which, in turn, is observed by the world at large. What we create in our lives begins as a basic image in our minds. Visualize the way you want to walk, stand, move. In Body Maintenance, visualization is an important next step after learning the exercises. On a superficial level, many of the exercises appear fairly simple. However, how you physically position your arms or legs is only part of the process. It is necessary, even when working certain muscles, that you are equally focused on the rest of your body. Where are your feet? Are you holding your head in the right way? Is your body properly aligned?

Initially this can seem quite difficult; using visualization techniques can be enormously helpful. By understanding how your body *should* feel, it becomes easier to assume the correct position.

Visualization is one of the best methods to bridge the gap between mind and body. By creating mental pictures that correspond to what you are trying to do physically, you will, in time, develop a level of body awareness that is unique to Pilates-based exercises.

Basic Visualization Techniques

Anybody can learn to visualize. Start by relaxing, as a still mind helps to conjure up images.

Start by gathering your thoughts. Try to forget about external influences like work, or things you need to do. Remember, this is *your* time.

Focus on your breathing by taking slow, deep breaths. This can instantly help you to feel calm because it promotes soothing alpha brainwaves. You can add a few gentle stretches. Once you feel sufficiently relaxed, you can start your exercises.

As you perform each exercise, concentrate on how each part of your body feels. With each one, think of a specific picture. For example, if you try to envision yourself walking effortlessly through a cloud, concentrate clearly on how this feels. Do your feet feel relaxed, warm and comfortable? Are your arms hanging loosely by your sides? Where is your head? Thinking of these images will help you to relax into the correct position.

Let your mind create each image with as much intensity as possible, so you can almost feel it. This will help you with your exercises as, once you recall a familiar picture, all you will need to do is focus on it and your body will automatically respond.

Even when not exercising, using these visualization techniques can help bring about permanent changes. You can use visualization to help you walk, stand and sit in the correct way.

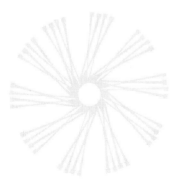

Essentials

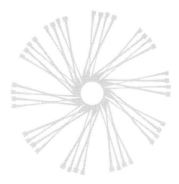

Because Body Maintenance is a very precise system of exercise, it is important that you first become acquainted with the basic principles. This groundwork will help you fully understand what you are doing. There are six essential guidelines to follow.

1 BREATHING

It is important to be aware of the relationship between breath and movement. Emphasized in dance but rarely addressed at the gym, breathing correctly is fundamental to Pilates. For most exercises in this book, you should breathe out at the point of effort.

As oxygen nourishes the brain and the body, it is crucial to breathe deeply, right down into the lower lobes of your lungs, not just using the upper chest. Most people are stronger on one side of their body than on the other, looser on one side and tighter on the other. Pilates uses breathing and exercise to create balance in the body.

Breathing deeply, you're working from the inside out, energizing and replenishing large areas of your body. It is as spiritual as it is physical. Breathing into a tight area that is being stretched after a long time is rejuvenating. Think of breathing as a form of liberation.

2 CONTROL

'Control' in this instance means that the correct part of the body is used in each exercise. By focusing on a particular muscle group, you are able to minimize the stress and involvement of other parts of the body. Doing an abdominal curl without this kind of focus and attention, for example, often leads to straining of the neck, shoulders and hip flexors, instead of working the abdominal muscles.

All exercises must be done slowly and in a meditative fashion. Control and precision are key. Your mind must concentrate on what you're doing. It is preferable to do 10 repetitions in a thoughtful and regulated way than to do a 100 mechanically, using only momentum. When working with free weights, for example, you should be able to use internal resistance rather than using your shoulders or snapping your elbows. Similarly, in the pelvic tilts you should be able to feel one vertebra at a time. Pilates is about being sensitive to your body.

People often make what is a simple exercise into something that is torturous, thus creating distortion and tension. Proper control makes each exercise efficient by concentrating on each muscle group, while keeping the rest of the body relaxed and aligned.

3 CENTRING

Pilates encourages the development of one strong, core area that controls the rest of the body and supplies it with energy. This core is the centre of your body: the continuous band between the bottom of your ribcage and across the line of your hipbones. The area's stomach and back muscles support your spine and internal organs, and keep you upright.

This central stability supports its various extensions – the arms, legs and head. Having a strong core means you can walk and run without discomfort or pain. Similarly, a strong centre results in a strong back, and backache can be alleviated by strengthening the core muscles.

Human beings were not originally designed to stand up straight. As gravity is constantly pulling us forward, it explains why so many people have problems associated with the neck and shoulders. We are basically defying nature, gravity and our initial body type by walking and standing upright.

4 FLOW

If any action feels quick, jerky or sharp, you can be sure that you are performing the exercise incorrectly. Every movement in Pilates originates from a strong centre and flows out in a slow, gentle, controlled manner. This warms the muscles, causing them to lengthen and open up the spaces between each vertebra in the spine, extending the body. The result is a longer, leaner look.

5 PRECISION

Performing Pilates with precision ensures that each movement is working the body in the correct manner. It is therefore important to read the instructions carefully before starting an exercise sequence. Make sure you are properly aligned, and pay attention to the 'Watchpoint' notes. This will ensure that you do not expend excess energy doing an exercise incorrectly.

6 CO-ORDINATION

Children run and bend naturally, but for most adults basic co-ordination is a major problem. When starting Body Maintenance, I have heard people say, 'I can't co-ordinate my breath with the movement. It's too much. I've got to concentrate too hard. I can't do it.' Many people have lost the ability to co-ordinate their bodies and minds as parts of the same working machine. The aim of Pilates is to retrain the neuromuscular connection between the brain and the body.

We all have the capability to be in touch with every part of our body, but we often don't use it. Those who have lost the use of their hands, for instance, have been known to train their feet to carry out many of the same functions. Yet for most of us, employing our feet in this way would seem impossible. If you don't utilize a part of your body, it atrophies. You have to think of co-ordination in much the same way.

By co-ordinating your breath and using a strong centre, getting your right arm and opposite (left) leg to work together without any difficulty is possible. The ability to react spontaneously is a result of the neuromuscular connection between brain and body. This is where the proprioceptive concept – the linking of mind and body – comes into play. Pilates enhances this sense of co-ordination in every exercise sequence through breath and precision.

Key Terms

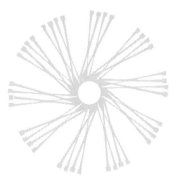

In Pilates and Body Maintenance there are certain key terms that are referred to over and over again. It will help if you understand these before you begin.

RELAXING

Many people associate relaxation with a feeling of 'letting go', of allowing muscles to slump. In the case of Pilates, to relax means to release tension in an area while still managing to maintain tone and control. When do you this, it should feel comfortable and natural.

NEUTRAL SPINE

Some positions will require you to keep your spine in 'neutral'. This means that you maintain the natural curve in your back. Thus, when you are lying down, do not press your back so hard into the floor that you lose the back's natural curve. Neither should you arch your back so that your lower back comes off the floor. Just lie there, breathe in and out naturally and allow your back to relax into the floor without pressing it in. This will allow your back to relax into its own natural, neutral position, which is slightly different for each person. Think of your body floating on a cloud.

THE CENTRE

In Body Maintenance, every exercise originates from the centre. The stomach muscles are the core to everything and they support the spine. It is important that you always remember to keep this area correctly aligned. This is particularly important when exercising the lower abdominals, as it is very easy to do the opposite of what you actually want. It is natural for the stomach to pull into the spine when you breathe in and to bulge out when you exhale. This is not what *you* want. You will have to try and reverse what the body wants to do unconsciously. As you breathe in, relax your stomach. As you exhale, pull your navel towards your spine, engaging the lower abdominal muscles. It is important to engage the stomach muscles when you breathe out.

THE FEET

You want your feet to remain relaxed when performing most of the exercises. If you are in doubt – relax your feet. Most people tense their feet too much. The result can be getting a cramp when they are exercising. (If you do get a cramp, use a foot-roller to ease away the tension.) A relaxed foot should feel comfortable, so that there is no tension or tightness. Whenever you flex your foot, do so by gently stretching out your heel then pulling the top of your foot as far as you can without straining. Take care not to tense your foot so that it feels strained.

THE NECK

It is important always to follow the neck instructions in these exercises very carefully. As this is a sensitive part of the body you do not want to put it under unnecessary strain while you are exercising. Body Maintenance often refers to keeping your neck long. This means adjusting your head into a position that lengthens your neck. When lying on your back for an exercise, the way you bring your head into alignment with the rest of your body is by moving the top of your skull and the base of your neck. Do not try to flatten your neck against the floor.

STRAIGHT ARMS AND LEGS

This common term in Body Maintenance means that your arms and legs should be relaxed and not locked. This is important to remember, particularly for the stretches. When an exercise requires you to stretch your arm or leg out straight, you should be careful not to overextend it, as this can cause the joints to lock.

Body Basics

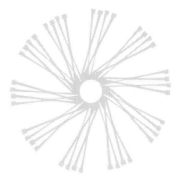

The main function of the skeletal system is to provide your body with support, protection and movement. Bones act as levers: when muscles pull on the bones, this causes parts of the body to move. Muscles are attached to the bones by tendons composed of tough, fibrous, non-elastic connective tissue. Body Maintenance focuses primarily on the main 25 bones that comprise the spinal column, consisting of:

• Seven cervical vertebrae in the neck

• Twelve thoracic vertebrae, articulating with the ribs in the thorax

• Five lumbar vertebrae in the lower back

• Four bones fused together into the coccyx at the base of the spine.

ONE VERTEBRA AT A TIME

This is one of the main principles that you should keep in mind whenever you are doing an exercise that involves rolling your body up and down on the ball. The idea is that you should roll up gradually so that you are lifting only one vertebra off the floor at a time. It is the same when you roll back down again. This takes some practice, and initially you will need to concentrate very carefully to ensure that you are doing it correctly.

MOVEMENTS

All movements involving the bones occur at the joints, thus enabling a variety of different postures. The more common ones you will come across in Body Maintenance are:

FLEXION which bends a limb or the spine, e.g. when bending the head forward onto the chest

EXTENSION which straightens a limb or the spine

HYPEREXTENSION which means bending back further than the vertical position, e.g. moving your head backwards so you can see the ceiling

ABDUCTION when you make a move away from the centre of the body, e.g. raising your arms horizontally sideways

ADDUCTION when you move towards the centre of your body, e.g. lowering your arms to your sides

INVERSION when something turns inwards, e.g. turning the sole of your foot inwards

ROTATION when the body turns on its axis either away from or towards the centre of the body

THE MUSCLES

Muscles are responsible for maintaining posture. Many muscles are attached by tendons to two articulating bones. A movement is created by muscles exerting a pull on these tendons, which move the bones at the joints. Therefore, most movements involve the use of several muscle groups. Muscles may also work in 'antagonistic' pairs – one muscle contracts to move the bone in one direction while the other muscle contracts to move it in another, like the calf and shin muscles which raise and lower the foot.

Each muscle has the ability to contract and shorten. It can be stretched when it is relaxed. Muscles also control internal functions such as pumping blood around the body and propelling food through the digestive system. There are hundreds of muscles in the body (of which 620 can be consciously controlled), all of which are involved in a wide range of functions.

The most important muscles you should be aware of for the purpose of Body Maintenance are:

TRAPEZIUS in the back of the neck, running down to the shoulders.
Action – extends the head.

LEVATOR SCAPULAE at the back and sides of the neck, running into the shoulders.
Action – lifts the shoulder blades and shoulders.

DELTOID on top of the shoulders and upper arms.
Action – moves the arm backwards and forwards.

BICEPS at the front of the arms.
Action – moves the arms.

TRICEPS at the back of the arms.
Action – moves the arms.

GLUTEUS MAXIMUS forms the buttocks.
Action – raises the body, used in running and jumping.

GLUTEUS MINIMUS in the buttocks.

Action – rotates the thigh laterally, maintains balance, used in walking and running.

SARTORIUS crosses the front of the thigh from the lateral to medial side.

Action – flexes the hip and knee, as when sitting cross-legged.

SEMITENDINOSUS (HAMSTRINGS) down the posterior medial side of the thigh.

Action – extends the thigh, flexes the leg at the knee.

QUADRICEPS EXTENSOR on the front of the thigh.

Action – opposite movement to hamstrings.

EXTERNAL OBLIQUE extends laterally down the side of the abdomen.

Action – compresses the abdomen, twists the trunk.

INTERNAL OBLIQUE extends laterally down the side of the front of the abdomen.

Action – compresses the abdomen, twists the trunk, works with the external oblique.

RECTUS ABDOMINIS runs down the entire length of the front of the abdomen (divided into four sections).

Action – an important muscle for maintaining posture, drawing the front of the pelvis forward.

TRANSVERSE ABDOMINIS runs laterally across the abdomen.
Action – compresses the abdomen.

ERECTOR SPINAE found medially on the posterior surface of the neck, thorax and abdomen.
Action – extends the spine and holds the body upright.

LATISSIMUS DORSI runs down the back of the lower thorax and lumbar region.
Action – draws the shoulders downwards and backwards, adducts and rotates the arms, helps pull the body up.

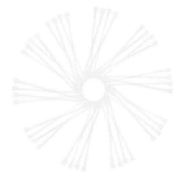

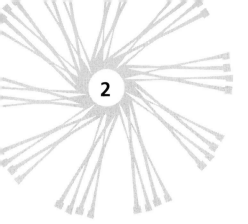

2

Body Awareness

Preparation: What you should know before you start to exercise

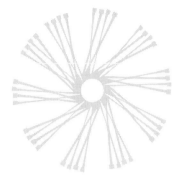

Before you begin *10-Minute Pilates with the Ball*, try this simple preliminary body awareness exercise:

Standing or sitting, close your eyes. Take a few deep breaths, then, starting with your head, slowly direct your focus down through your whole body. Visualize each part of your body as you imagine steering the flow of energy through it from part to part.

Visualize your eyes, ears, mouth, down your shoulders, arms and hands.

Visualize your chest, back, abdomen, hips, pelvic area, upper legs, knees, lower legs, ankles and feet.

As you visit each area, try to build up a mental picture of how it looks and feels. Spend a few seconds on each part. Move your head gently, shrug your shoulders. Gently move your stomach, tailbone and hips. Concentrate on the sensation as you do this. Which areas feel most comfortable and relaxed? Are certain areas tight and constricted?

Now repeat, seated on the ball in the perfect posture position (see page 46). Make sure to hold on to something, if your eyes are closed.

Do this for a few minutes each day. It will help you to become more aware of your body when you are ready to begin to exercises.

The *10-Minute Pilates with a Ball* exercises require total concentration and focus. It is therefore important to find a time and place to do them where you know you will not be disturbed or interrupted. Find a corner of your home where you will not be distracted, and use it as a retreat. This helps to get you in the right frame of mind. You can do this by thinking 'This is my time, I am creating a space in my own environment, to work on my body for myself.'

WHEN TO EXERCISE

You can perform these exercises at any time of day. Choose the early evening to help you unwind and loosen tight muscles after a busy day. If you find it difficult to start your mornings with energy, a 10-minute session early in the day may be just what you need.

CLOTHES

Choose items you can exercise in comfortably, such as a T-shirt or leotard top worn with leggings or shorts. Avoid clothing that will restrict your movements. Cotton and other natural fabrics are cooler than man-made ones. Your feet can be bare or you can wear socks. If you are concerned about slipping, put on a pair of trainers. Remove any jewellery that could get in the way. Remember, the ball is unstable, so make sure you feel secure.

EQUIPMENT

Create an adequate space in the room where you will exercise. Your surroundings could be cleared of clutter, or furniture could be moved to enable you to move freely. Check the floor for pins or other sharp objects which could injure you or damage the Physio Ball. Keep away from hot radiators, etc.

It is essential to use a mat or padded surface for when you lie on the floor, to protect your spine and prevent any bruising. It is probably worth investing in a proper sports mat. Alternatively, you can work on a folded, synthetic blanket. Always make sure the furniture is secure. If an exercise indicates a couple of light weights and you don't have any, you can substitute tins of beans or plastic bottles of water.

If possible, try to exercise in front of a full-length mirror. This will enable you to check what you are doing.

WHICH EXERCISES?

It is important always to start your core exercise routine with the seated ball exercises before moving on to the floor exercises, because this way you will be working from a strong centre. This is true even when you are exercising your arms or legs, as everything is controlled from the centre. As well as doing some basic abdominal work, you should follow strengthening exercises with the relevant stretches. You can then alternate upper and lower bodywork each day.

SEQUENCE OF EXERCISES

1 At the beginning, do all the seated ball exercises that have to do with balance and shoulder releases.

2 Move on to the pelvic tilt and abdominal exercises.

3 Follow with the back exercises.

4 Do leg exercises and stretches.

5 Finish with upper body exercises and stretches.

Read all the instructions carefully. Always remember the breathing instructions.

Use your own judgement. After starting with the pelvic tilt and abdominal exercises, continue to add a little each time as you feel more comfortable. If you feel discomfort in your back during any particular exercise, this means you have insufficient core strength to do it.

The following safety rules will help:

- Always do stretches after the relevant strengthening exercises.

- Do not attempt to do too much too soon. Increase the repetitions gradually.

- Always stop if you feel nauseous, fatigued or extremely breathless.

- If you have any chest pains (especially when accompanied by pain in the arms, neck, shoulders and jaw) – stop exercising immediately and seek medical help.

- Check with your doctor if exercise leaves you unnaturally tired.

- The neck is a sensitive area. If you cannot remember whether you have worked this area or not, it is better not to do any further repetitions.

- Always make sure that there is something you can hold on to for support when doing the balancing exercises.

- If you experience back pain – stop.

- If your muscles start shaking – stop.

- Drink plenty of fluids after exercising, especially when it is hot.

It is a good idea to consult your doctor before embarking on any new exercise programme. A pre-exercise check-up is strongly advised if you are over 40 or have not been exercising regularly. Always seek the advice of a specialist if you have a medical condition, are pregnant or have any chronic joint problems.

SIZE AND PRESSURE

Physio Balls are size-related. On the correct-sized ball for your height you should be able to sit with your hips and knees at a 90-degree angle. Anyone below 5ft 8in (173cm) tall should use a 55-cm ball. Anyone 5ft 8in to 5 ft 9in (173cm to 176cm) should use a 65-cm ball. Having said this, I would recommend that most people, except men over 6ft (182cm), should get a 55-cm ball, because for most of the exercises, like press-ups over the ball, you will want the smaller-sized ball.

Pump up the ball so that it feels firm and solid. If it feels soggy, you need to keep pumping, which is best done at a garage forecourt air-pump or by using a foot pump at home.

PRECAUTIONS

The ball should not be placed anywhere near sharp objects or near heat. Do not allow children to play with it. Do not exercise wearing sharp objects like buckles or belts. Foremost, you need to remember that the ball is an unstable surface, so at the beginning of every exercise it is important to start near something or someplace you can actually hold on to. This is particularly important if you are pregnant or you have any problems with instability in your spine or hips, or if you feel you have reached a certain age where you do not have good balance.

Breathing

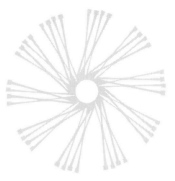

Correct breathing is an essential facet of Pilates. As you breathe properly you will find it becomes much easier to exercise. The problem is that most people don't breathe deeply enough. Breathing slowly and deeply is very energizing, as it ensures there is sufficient oxygen circulating throughout the body.

It may sound obvious, but be careful not to hold your breath when you exercise. It's better to breathe incorrectly than not at all.

Practise this exercise before you start any stomach work.

BASIC BREATHING EXERCISE

- Seated on the ball, knees hip-width apart, arms hanging loosely beside and slightly in front of your body, feel relaxed, head 'floating' upwards, relaxed on your neck.

- Place one hand on your stomach and very gently breathe in through your nose. Feel your lungs fill with oxygen and slowly expand and relax your stomach.

- With one finger on your pubic bone and one on your navel, try to shorten that gap as you breathe out, and flatten your stomach to your spine without moving the ball.

- Breathe in again and feel that gap slightly expand.

- Breathe out. Imagine there is a piece of string or an elastic band that links your pubic bone to your navel. Feel it very gently pulling up and in. This will make all three sets of stomach muscles work, including your oblique muscles, which will tighten your waist.

Try always to breathe slowly and deeply. One of the main rules of Pilates is to breathe out on the point of effort. If in doubt, particularly on the stretches – breathe naturally.

When you breathe in, your stomach gently expands. It should not, however, swell in an exaggerated way. Try and think of your ribcage expanding gently to the sides so that you're not just breathing into your throat and upper chest.

You may feel dizzy when you first start to breathe properly at the start of this exercise programme. This is because you are taking in more oxygen than normal, as you are breathing more deeply, which can make you feel light-headed.

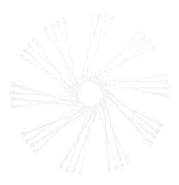

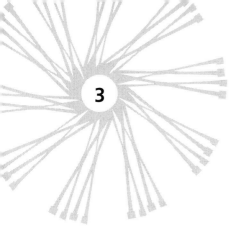

3

Pilates with the Ball

First Movements

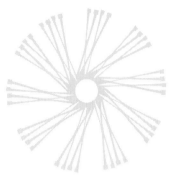

Sitting Properly

Seated on the ball, your tailbone heavy and both feet evenly placed on the floor, hip-width apart, try to be in contact from your centre directly down through your feet into the floor. You are going to channel your energies from this centre out through the crown of your head. Your shoulders and arms are relaxed. Your tailbone will drop and your abdominals will naturally pull back towards your spine. Try to think of your head sitting naturally on top of your shoulders, neither pushing it forward nor pulling it back.

Watchpoint: If you force your shoulders back, and your lower back arches away from the ball, you know your shoulders are still too rounded for you to maintain this position and be anatomically correct.

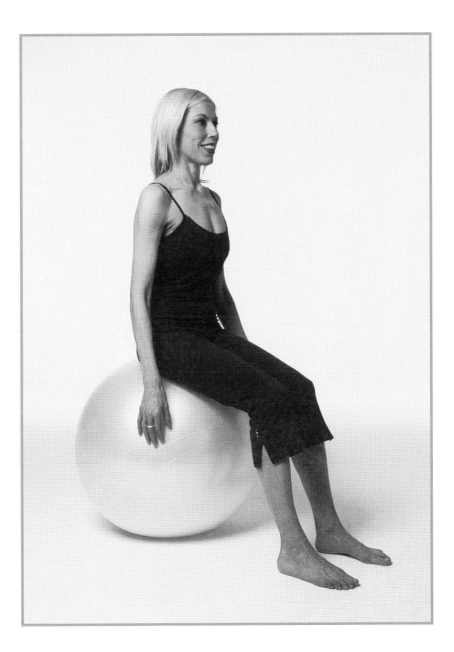

Pilates with the Ball

Double Shoulder Lifts

Sitting as above, squeeze both shoulders up to your ears. Make sure your hands are dangling loosely by your sides. Repeat 10 times.

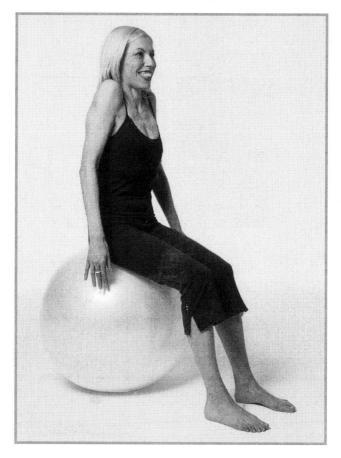

 Watchpoint: It is important not to lock your elbows or stick your chin forward.

Single Shoulder Lifts

These relax the shoulders and neck.

Sit comfortably on the ball with your arms relaxed at your sides. Breathe in, and slowly squeeze your right shoulder up to your right ear. Relax it down. Repeat with the other shoulder. Do this to a count of four up, four down. Don't move your head.

Repeat 10 times, alternating shoulders.

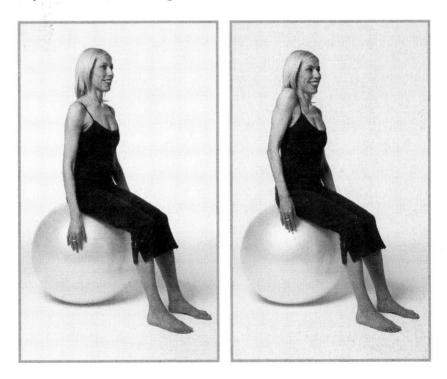

Shoulder Circles

Assume the same position as above. Place your hands on your shoulders and, very gently, circle both arms forward.

Repeat 10 times.

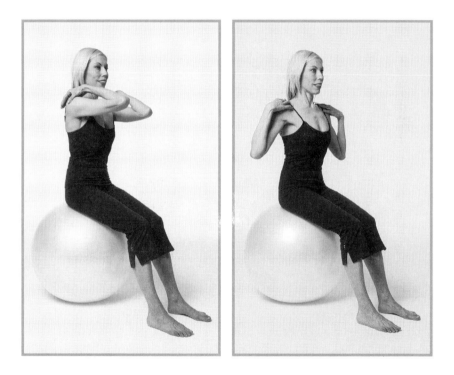

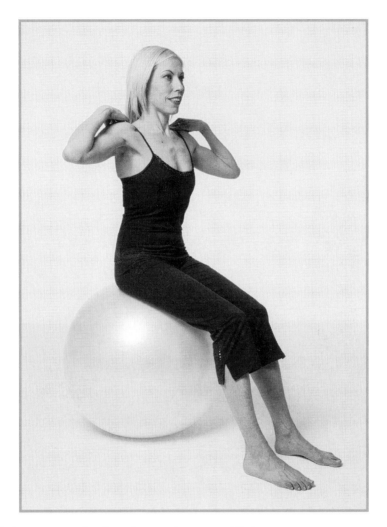

Circle your arms backwards – again, repeat 10 times.

If this feels uncomfortable, you may have tight wrists: try circling your shoulders with your arms hanging at your sides.

Foot Lifts

Seated on the ball, you can either have your fingers on your abdomen or allow your arms to hang naturally beside you. As you breathe in, your abdomen gently softens or expands into your fingers. As you breathe out, very gently let one foot float off the floor, feeling the connection of your navel to your spine. Place the foot down and ensure you have even pressure through both feet again. Then lift the other leg. Co-ordination is very important here. Start off Foot Lifts very slowly; eventually you will be able to do them faster so the interchange emanates from a stable pelvis and a strong abdomen.

Initially the change from one leg to the other might feel unstable, as you don't have the core strength to co-ordinate alternate leg lifts automatically. The feet should float off the floor.

Repeat for 10 lifts on each leg, alternating each time.

Watchpoint: If you lift your feet too high, you will lose balance and wobble on the ball, as well as lose that postural alignment. Your tailbone will tuck underneath and your back will curl. Start with the ball close to something you can hold on to, like a chair if you are worried about your balance.

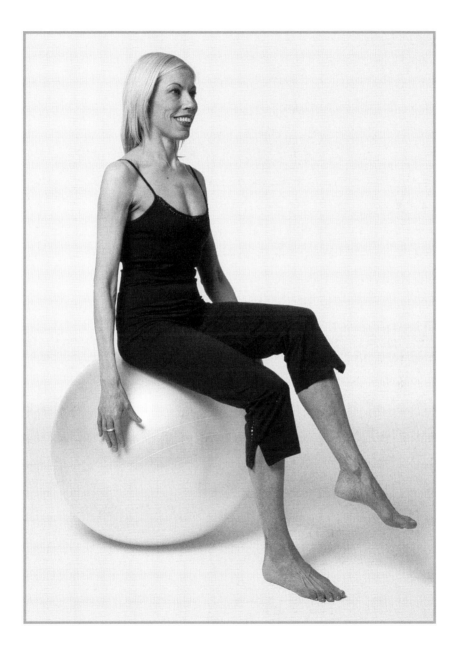

Abdominals

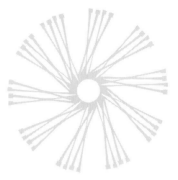

Pelvic Tilt

The pelvic tilt is a preparation exercise that warms up the back. It's a good starting point, whatever part of the programme you plan to do.

If you have high blood pressure, do not hold your breath in any of the bent-knee exercises. Keep your feet on the ball, knees and ankles in line, no pinching in the front of the hip and don't be too close to the ball.

Lie on your back with your knees bent and parallel, about hip-width apart with your feet on the ball supported against a wall. Your arms should be resting at your sides, with relaxed shoulders and palms facing the floor. This helps to lengthen your neck.

Breathe in, then breathe out and gently relax your back into the floor, your tailbone weighted on the mat. When you do this, do not press your back too strongly to the ground so that you lose your natural curve. Do not allow your back to arch to the point that it lifts off the floor. You want to maintain a neutral spine position, which is slightly different for each person. There is no point in trying to force your back down. Try very hard not to tense your buttock muscles during this exercise.

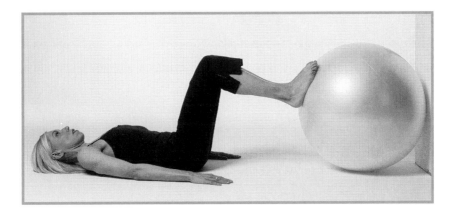

As you breathe out, gently tilt your pelvis forward and roll your lower back off the floor – one vertebra at a time, as you 'peel' your back off the mat until you are just below your shoulder blades. If you feel your ribs sticking forward or your neck shortening, you'll know you've gone too far.

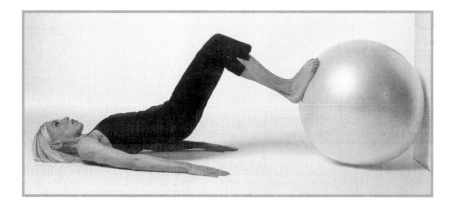

Breathe in, keeping your neck long, and very slowly roll all the way down, breathing out, until your tailbone reaches the floor. Keep your feet relaxed on the ball and imagine your toes 'lengthening' away. Do approximately 10 repetitions.

Watchpoint: Keep your legs parallel to each other, and grip your bottom as little as possible.

There is a good chance you will feel this contraction in your calf and hamstrings. Don't worry about this unless it is really uncomfortable. If this is the case, skip this exercise.

A more difficult version of this exercise is to have your elbows on the floor and rest back on them, palms off the floor. This is harder because you have a less stable base throughout the upper body. Don't be tempted to push too high.

When you become more confident, complete the pelvic tilts with the ball unsupported.

Preparation for Abdominals

This is a preparation for the abdominal exercises. It will wake up your stomach muscles and prepare you for the more difficult exercises.

Secure the ball against a solid surface. Lie on the floor with your feet on the ball, with a relaxed back and long neck, without tucking your pelvis under. Take either a small cushion or folded towel and place it between your thighs.

Very gently breathe in through your nose. As you breathe out, feel your stomach muscles pulling down to the floor. Think of them pulling up and into your spine. Hold your breath and count to four. Squeeze the towel or cushion with your thighs, contracting your deep internal muscles. You can put your fingers on your stomach if you wish so that you can feel the muscles you are working.

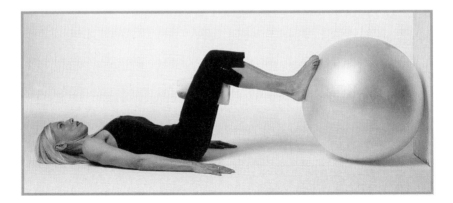

As you breathe in through your nose, feel your stomach gently expand into your fingers. As you breathe out, feel your stomach pull away from your fingers. Feel your lower abdominal muscles working. Think of working on the transverse and the rectus abdominus muscles first, and the obliques second.

Repeat 10 times.

Watchpoint: Don't let your pelvis lift off the floor. This will 'shorten' your neck. Watch that your stomach doesn't 'bloat'. Instead, make sure that on the point of relaxation – when you breathe in – your stomach gently expands. As you breathe out you should feel your stomach pull up and in, away from the pubic bone.

Most people naturally want to breathe in and pull their stomach muscles in – this is a mistake. As you breathe in, you gently soften the muscles as they flow out into your fingers. As you breathe out, the stomach pulls away from your fingers. Think of it as pulling 'up and in'. This will help you focus on your lower abdominals – strengthening and toning that area.

Working the Lower Abdominal Muscles

Lie in the same position as above, knees bent, legs together. You can place your hands on your hipbones. This helps to stabilize your pelvis.

Very gently breathe in and let your knees open to shoulder-width apart, making a small 'V' shape.

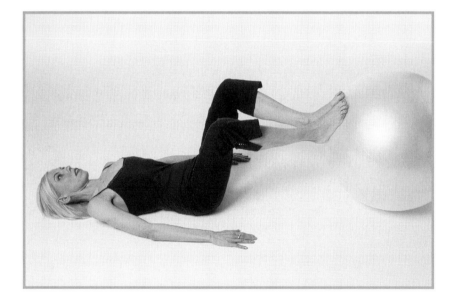

As you breathe out, feel the resistance. Bring your legs back together, focusing through your inner thighs as a passive resistance, breathing out and pulling your stomach in.

Repeat 10 times.

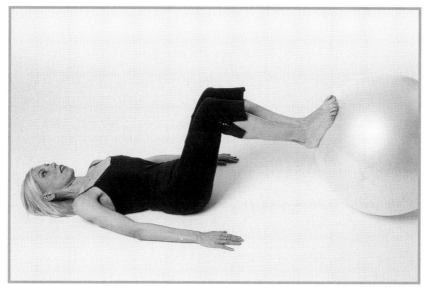

 Watchpoint: Think of the muscles between your navel and your pubic bone as a fan. As you inhale and your knees open to the side, the fan opens. As you exhale, the muscles tighten and the fan closes. Don't press your back into the mat.

Working the Lower Abdominal Muscles 2

This slightly harder version of the previous exercise is very straightforward. Interlace your hands behind your head (this will help prevent you from straining the muscles in your neck). Slide them high up behind your skull. Do not let them slip to your neck. Keep your thumbs on either side of your spine. Don't stick your chin out.

Lift your elbows so that you can just see them out of the corner of your eye without moving your head. When you can see your elbows peripherally you know that your arms are in the right place.

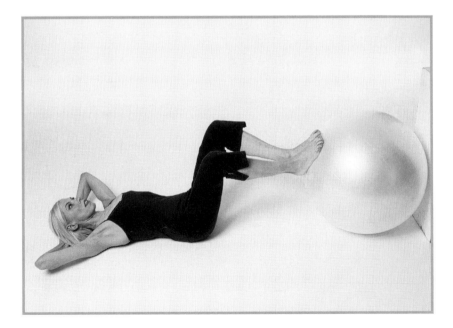

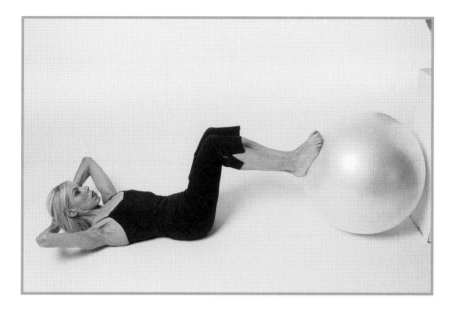

Very gently exhale and 'float' your head and shoulders off the mat. As you lift, squeeze your legs together, inhale and lower your head and shoulders, opening your legs again.

Repeat 10 times.

 Watchpoint: As you lift your head your focus shouldn't change, so you don't shorten your neck. If you shorten your neck, you may tip your pelvis. This makes it very hard to work your lower abdominal muscles. You may also place a strain on your lower back and your body will be incorrectly aligned.

Basic Abdominal Curl

This exercise uses exactly the same position as the previous exercise, although your feet and knees should be hip-width apart. All the same rules apply. Keeping your feet on the ball, lift your elbows up to where you can see them in your peripheral vision. Keep looking at the ceiling and gently breathe in through your nose. Relax your abdomen, but do not 'bloat' it out.

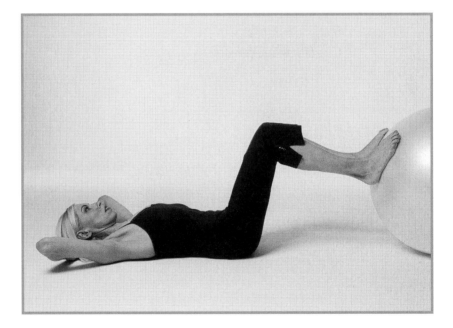

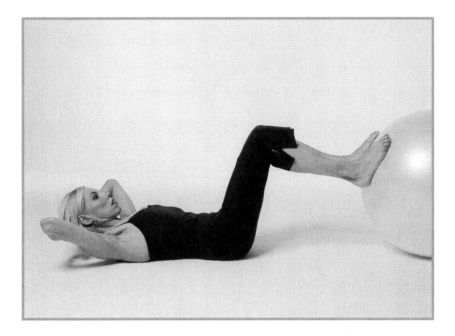

As you breathe out, gently lift your head and shoulders off the mat. Only go as high as you can. Do not strain your neck to hold the position.

Breathe in as you go back down again.

 Watchpoint: As you breathe out, imagine that a piece of string is pulling you up from the pubic bone and under your rib cage. Pause until all three sets of abdominal muscles go 'up and in', and flatten.

Straight Leg Lifts

Lie on your back with your hands beside you and your calves on the ball, keeping your legs comfortably externally rotated in the hip socket.

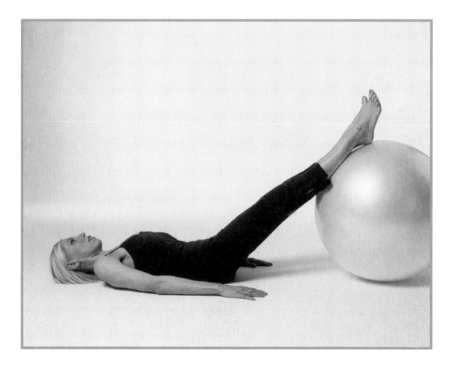

As you breathe out, lift your left leg, pulling up through the inside thigh, pull-ing in through the lower abdominals.

Breathe in as you lower your leg. Breathe out and lift your right leg.

Do not lift too high. Only lift as high as you feel comfortable with the ham-strings in the back of your leg. Placing your hands on your hips will ensure you don't lift too high, as you will otherwise pinch into your hip.

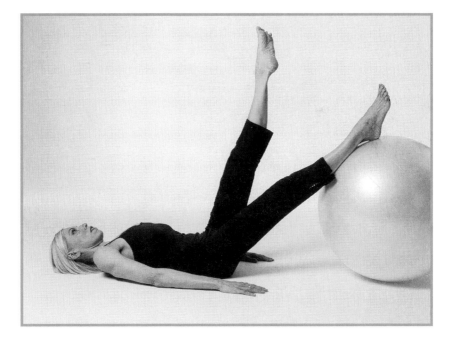

To make this exercise harder, do exactly the same routine but add a small sit-up into the lift, making it a more co-ordinated exercise.

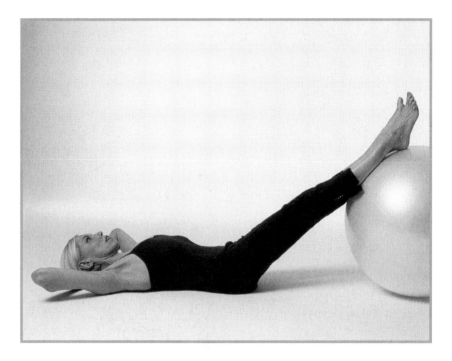

10-Minute Pilates with the Ball

As you breathe out and lift your leg, curl forward in a similar way to the earlier abdominal curl exercise, and breathe in as you lower both your leg and upper body.

Do a maximum of 10 repetitions of both exercises, five on each leg, alternating each time.

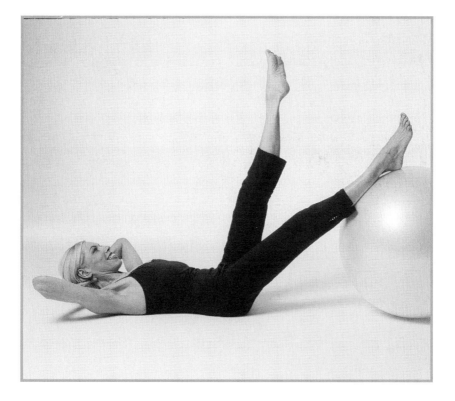

Lower Abdominal Exercise

Lie in the starting position as for the abdominal preparation exercises (page 58). The ball is unsupported in this exercise. The feet are comfortably positioned on the ball, with your hips and knees in line, and hands on your hips. Everybody tends to reverse this exercise, so it is very important to concentrate. It is a small movement.

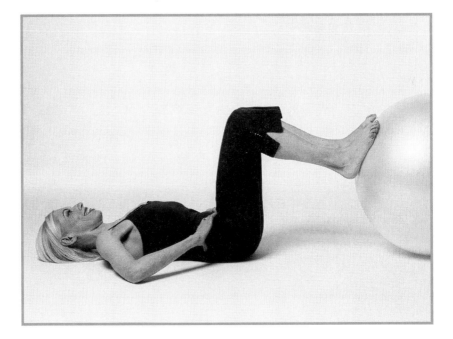

As you breathe in, push the ball away from you – about half a metre or a foot.

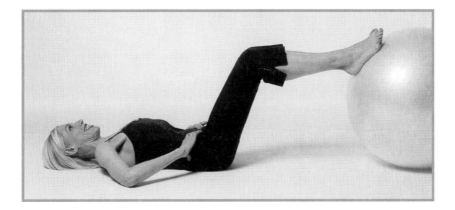

As you breathe out, draw the ball towards you using your lower abdominals, particularly the transverse abdominus, which are between your hip bones (the ones you use in the fanning exercise).

Two common mistakes can happen: if you push the ball too far away, your back will arch and you will feel uncomfortable as you breathe in. If as you breathe out you draw the ball in too far, you will pinch your hips. Your hands will tell you if you've come too far.

Repeat 10 times.

The next two exercises are the most advanced in the abdominal sequence. If you have any lower back problems at all, I suggest that you leave these exercises until you feel strong enough.

Advanced Abdominals

Lying on your back with the ball between your calves, keep your knees relaxed. You want the ball to be reasonably close to you. If you feel your lower back arching, bring the ball closer. However, you don't want the ball so close that your bottom leaves the floor. It is difficult to recommend exactly the position of your legs, because this varies from person to person. You want to feel secure, with your lower back supported.

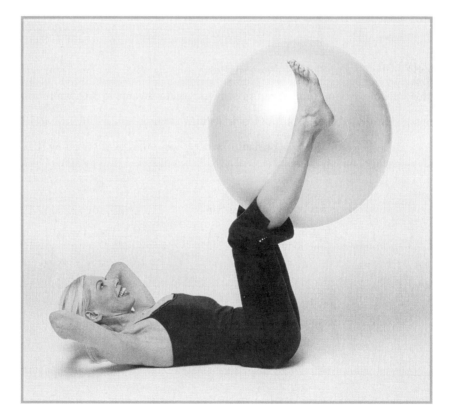

Leaving the ball suspended in the air between your calves, the exercise is similar to the basic abdominal curl.

Breathe out and curl forward, engaging your navel to your spine.

Breathe in as you lower yourself.

If this exercise is very demanding you can start with 4 repetitions and slowly build up to 10.

Watchpoint: When lifting your legs, bend your knees as you place the ball between your calves. When you lower your legs, take the ball from your calves with your hands and then bend your knees as you put your feet back on the ground.

Never lift from or lower the ball to the ground using your legs. Take the ball in your hands and 'position' the ball on the way up, and remove the ball before returning your feet to the ground.

Advanced Abdominals 2

The last exercise for the abdominals is again a challenging one, working the obliques, which are the muscles that support your waist. It is a great waist-toning exercise.

Lying on your side in a straight line, position the ball between your calves. Bring your legs slightly forwards and ensure you do not have an arch in your lower back. Breathe in.

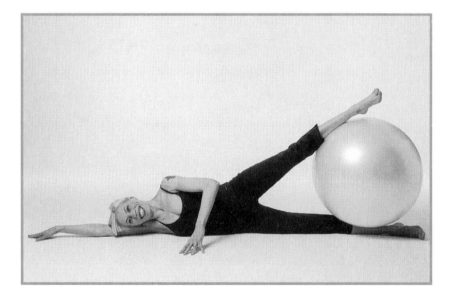

As you breathe out, lift your legs off the ground, pulling your stomach in. As you lift your legs, you want to draw the 'underneath' part of your waist off the mat. If your underneath waist and hip are sinking into the mat, you

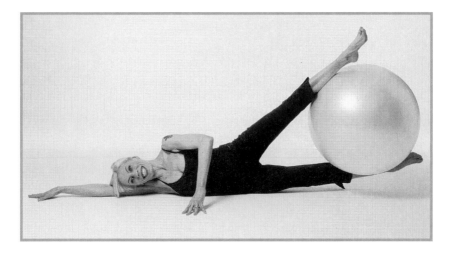

have lifted too far. If you have any discomfort in your lower back at all, bring your legs further forwards.

Do 10 repetitions, alternating sides.

If you have any worries about your back at all, build up to this exercise (and the previous one) over a period of weeks or months.

Watchpoint: If this is the first time you are doing this exercise, even possibly the first four times, I suggest that you lie on your side with your back against a wall so you can feel your middle back supported by the wall. Having your middle back supported will give you a clearer proprioceptive sense of spinal integrity.

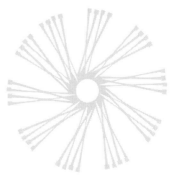

Strengthening Your Back

Cat Stretch

This exercise will release your lower back and stretch out your shoulders. The Cat Stretch is essential for spinal health, as it works equally on flexion and extension, both essential functions for a healthy spine.

Support the ball against the wall. Kneel as far away as you can while still resting your palms on the ball. Your weight should be distributed evenly through both knees. Your hips should be in line with your knees.

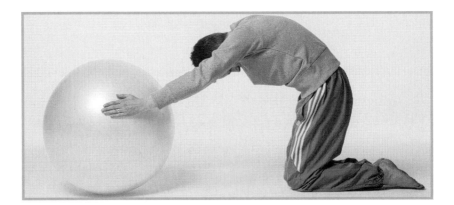

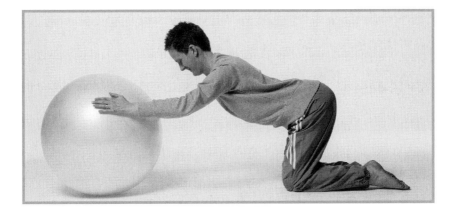

Breathe out, curl your chin into your chest, stomach into your spine, and stretch out your lower back, from the inside out, drawing all your internal organs into your spine. You get the blood flowing as you open your spine, and this will counteract the effects of being seated for long periods of time.

As you breathe in, press your chest down, your bottom up and gently lengthen your neck and head, stretching out tight shoulders and the upper thoracic spine.

This counts as one repetition. Repeat 10 times.

 Watchpoint: If you feel your neck crunching or your vocal cords contracting you've taken your head too far back. There should be no discomfort in your neck.

Make sure your feet stay on the floor.

Kneeling Arm and Leg Stretch

This exercise helps improve balance, stabilizes the pelvis and strengthens the spine and abdominal muscles.

Rest the ball under your stomach with your feet on floor, legs straight and hands in front of you shoulder-width apart. The spine is neutral and stomach gently in.

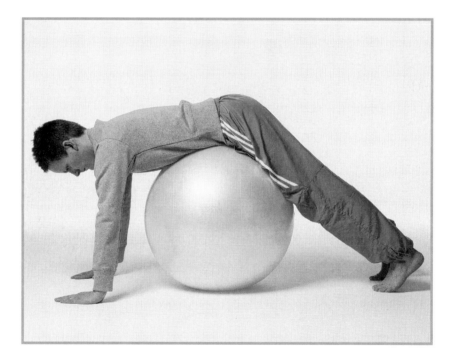

Breathe in and, as you breathe out, let your right arm and left leg gently float away. Don't lift too high or your hip will leave the ball. To avoid this, position something like a kitchen roll across the base of your spine. If you lift too high, it will fall off. Keep your pelvis neutral, so that you don't tilt from side to side. Keep looking at the same point on the floor, so that you don't shorten your neck. Relax back into the starting position.

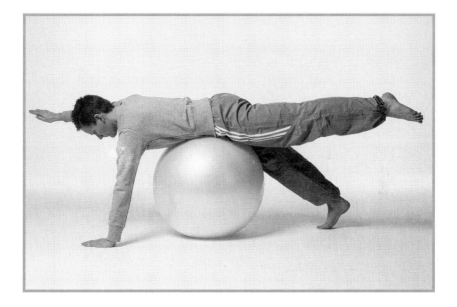

Repeat, alternating arms and legs, for 10 repetitions.

 Watchpoint: If this exercise feels too difficult at the onset, you can start by lifting one arm or one leg only, rather than both together at the same time.

Back Extension

You may feel more stable wearing trainers for this exercise. Have your feet based against a secure surface like a wall. Position your legs hip-width apart, securely against the wall. Relax over the ball with your hips against the ball and your hands behind your back. Breathe in.

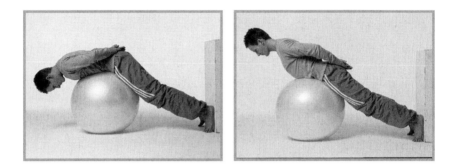

As you breathe out, curl forward on flexion, pulling your stomach in. Extend to a straight back, pause, then breathe in.

Breathe out and reverse the curl. This is similar to a cat stretch.

Watchpoint: As you curl forward, keep looking at the same point unless you have a very flexible spine.

You may feel your hamstring tightening a certain amount, but you don't want to stabilize it by gripping your buttocks. Keep the buttocks muscles relaxed.

Ensure that your shoulders are also relaxed, and do not lift them up to your ears. Keep your head and neck in line. If you lift your head too far and take it behind you, you will shorten the muscles in your neck. You will know if you are doing the exercise incorrectly if you feel pinching in your lower back or in your neck.

If you go too far and your stomach bulges out, you will not be strengthening your back but weakening it.

The Swan – Advanced Back Exercise

Start in the same position as the previous back exercise, but move away from the wall. Position the ball under your hips and breathe in. As you breathe out, tip the ball forward so you are resting on the palms of your hands, your legs in the air behind you. Breathe in.

Breathe out, reverse the movement, and let your feet come on to the floor and your arms float above your head, shoulder-width apart. This movement counts as one repetition.

Start with four and build up to a maximum of 10.

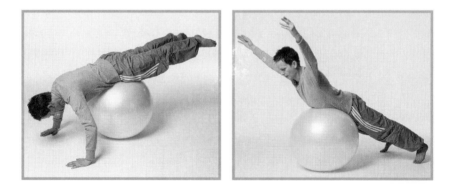

Watchpoint: In my studio I call this the Flying Swan. Obviously it is a very demanding exercise for the abdominals and the spine, but more importantly you have to be secure in your balance to stabilize the ball under your pelvis as you move forward and back on the ball.

Many people wear trainers for this exercise to stabilize their legs so they don't slip.

As with all back exercises, the stomach is the instigator of the movement. As you breathe out your stomach goes in, the shoulders are relaxed and the buttocks are not tensed.

Make sure that as your stomach goes in, your pelvis relaxes back. As you breathe in, don't grip your bottom.

Keep your legs straight. If you bend your knees, the exercise won't be as effective.

Keep your shoulders relaxed, stomach in, legs and arms straight. Your arms and legs should be at the same height, and should lift to the same height during the exercise.

Hip Roll (both legs)

Lie on your back with your feet on the ball, feet and legs together and your tailbone on the floor. Your ankles and knees should be in line with your hips, your feet relaxed. Breathe in.

As you breathe out, move your legs one way, your head the other way – your stomach should remain stable.

Breathe in and come back to the centre.

Repeat in the opposite direction.

 Watchpoint: The most important part of this exercise is that at no point should either shoulder blade leave the mat. Your knees should stay together as you move from side to side – this way one leg won't get longer than the other. It is very natural as you move from side to side to take the knees further than the ankles, but you want to keep them in line with your ankles – the movement is taken from the abdominals as the legs and the ball go from side to side.

This is a small movement. Do not let the ball take you further over than your abdominals can control the movement.

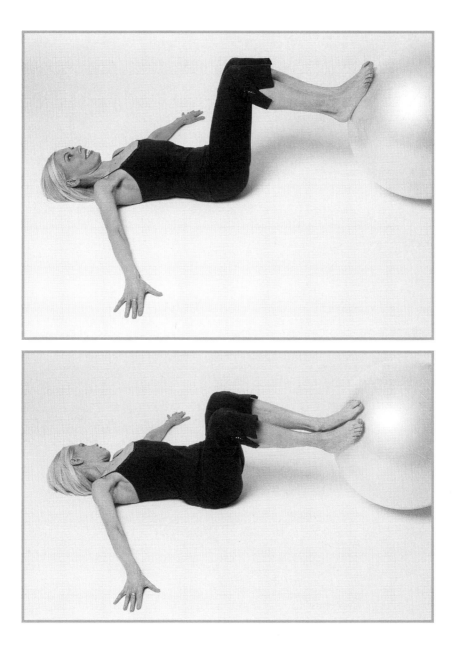

Toning and Stretching Your Legs

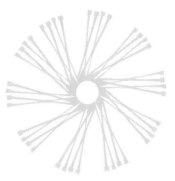

Inside Thigh Lift

This exercise will help tone your inner thighs. Lie on your side, either with your hand supporting your head or with your arm completely flat. If you choose to keep your arm flat, it may feel more comfortable to put a towel between your arm and ear. The other hand is in front of you. Your top leg should be forward, in front of your body, with your foot on the ball. The underneath leg needs to be slightly forward, with your foot gently flexed. Don't lock the knee, but pull up the muscles so that your leg is straight. If your legs are not straight, you'll be working your ankle and your foot too much.

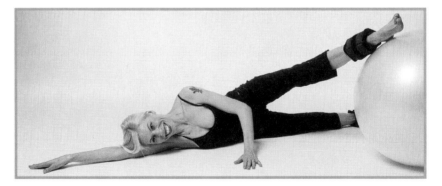

Breathe in and then, as you breathe out, lift your 'underneath' leg and hold. Then slowly lower it. Don't lift your leg too high. Think of your leg as going 'away', not up – you want to lengthen and strengthen your muscles, not have them contracted and tight. As you lift and breathe out, your stomach pulls in, just like in the earlier stomach exercises. The energy is through the heel, working your inside thigh. Do 10 on each side.

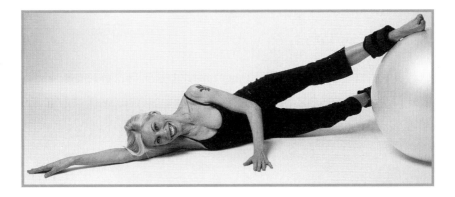

 Watchpoint: It's important to remember that, in all the leg exercises, the instigator is your stomach. This means you should feel your abdominal muscles working. The same applies to all the upper body exercises. Make sure your hips are stacked one on top of the other. You can use a wall to make sure your back is in the correct position. If in doubt, bring the underneath leg forward.

Inside Thigh Lift 2

Lie on your side as in the above exercise.

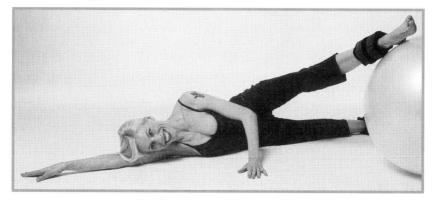

Breathe in and, as you breathe out, lift the underneath leg, bend the knee gently and then squeeze to straighten it. Keep your foot gently flexed, your knee unlocked, and your hips stacked on top of each other.

Do 10 repetitions, keeping your leg in the air the whole time.

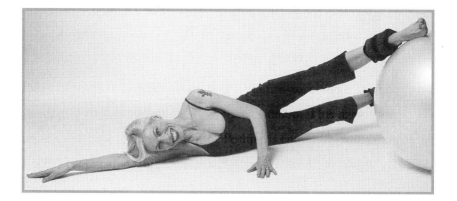

Bottom Toner

These next three exercises are all executed with your stomach on the ball. Lie on your front, position the ball comfortably between your ribs and hips, arms shoulder-width apart, neck in line, legs hip-width apart, feet on the floor and flexed for balance. Do not lock your elbows, and keep your wrists in line.

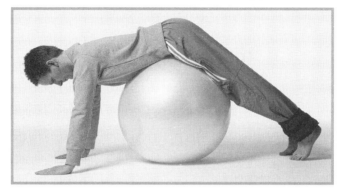

Keeping your foot softly flexed so as to engage the correct muscles, very gently breathe in, then breathe out and lift your leg. Then slowly bring it down, keeping the buttocks tightly gripped. Do 10 repetitions on each leg.

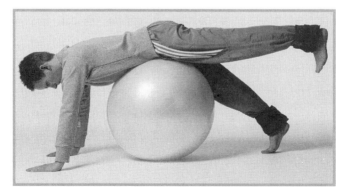

Bottom Toner 2

Assume the same position as the above exercise, still keeping your feet softly flexed.

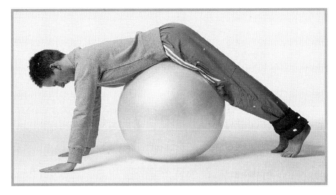

Breathe in, then very gently breathe out and lift both legs up. Slowly bring
them down, remembering to keep the buttocks gripped. Do 10 repetitions.

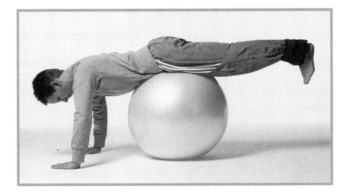

Bottom Toner 3

All the same rules apply as above. Starting in the same position, this time lift one leg off the floor to parallel with your hip, flexing your foot as you lift.

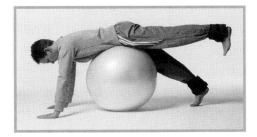

Bend at the knee so your ankle and knee are in line. Squeeze and lift the leg 10 times, keeping your hip on the ball so as not to distort your pelvis.

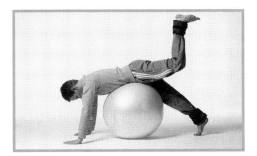

 Watchpoint: At no point in any of these exercises should your hipbones leave the ball. If you feel discomfort in your lower back, adjust your position slightly over the ball, alternatively do not lift your legs so high to begin with. Very occasionally people feel nauseous lying over a ball, so be aware of this.

Hamstring Toner and Strengthener

Lean forward over the ball with your hands firmly on the floor and your feet on the ground. Keep your shoulders relaxed. Breathe in and very gently 'grip' (tighten) your bottom. You should feel your stomach going in and your tailbone drop. Exhaling, raise your right leg and flex your foot.

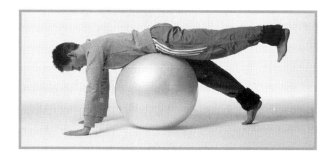

Then gently inhale and bend your leg, keeping your buttocks squeezed at all times. Exhale and straighten the leg, keeping it in the air for 10 repetitions, breathing in as you bend it, and out as you straighten it.

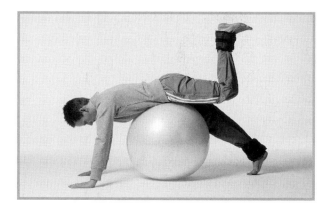

Standing Calf Stretch

Stand up straight using the ball as a support against a wall, hands comfortably apart. Take a step forward with your left leg and, leaning against the ball, bend the knee slightly and feel the stretch down through your right leg. Keep your right heel down. Do not bounce. Hold for 30 seconds. Repeat 4 times, alternating legs.

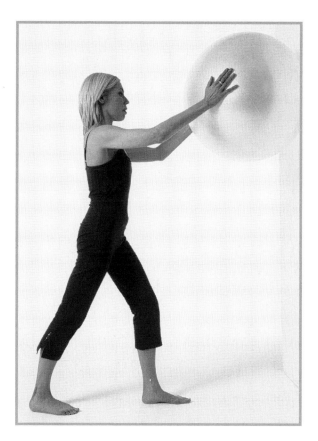

Back and Hip – Gluteal Stretch

This exercise will help to release your hips.

Lying on your back with your legs bent and feet resting on the ball, supported by a wall, very gently cross your left ankle over the right knee. Make sure it's the ankle, and not the toes. Use your left hand to press your left knee towards the ball, making sure your hips do not twist. Remember, you should feel a stretch only in the working leg. Hold for 30 seconds, change legs and repeat four times.

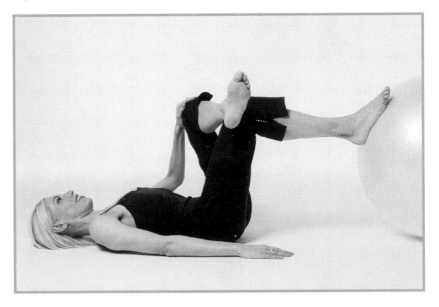

 Watchpoint: Make sure your tailbone stays on the floor.

Quadriceps Stretch

Kneel down on your right leg, keeping your back straight and with your hands resting on the ball supported by a wall. Extend your left leg, making sure that your heel is always in front of your knee. Gently pull your stomach in and lean back slightly, making sure you don't arch your back. Hold for 30 seconds. Repeat twice for each leg.

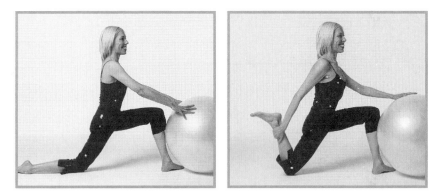

To make this exercise more challenging, take one hand off the ball and use it to take hold of your back ankle and draw it towards your bottom.

Watchpoint: If this stretch causes any pain in your knee or back, stop at once.

Lying Hamstring Stretch

For this exercise, most people need to place a towel beneath their head. Lie on your mat or towel.

Resting your feet on the ball supported by a wall, knees bent, make sure you have equal weight down through both feet. Your arms are beside you and your pelvis is in the neutral position. Very gently bend your left knee into your chest. Grasp the back of your thigh with your left hand. Grasp the back of your calf with your right hand and gently unfold, straightening that leg with a flexed foot, and ease the leg towards you, moving your left hand up to your calf.

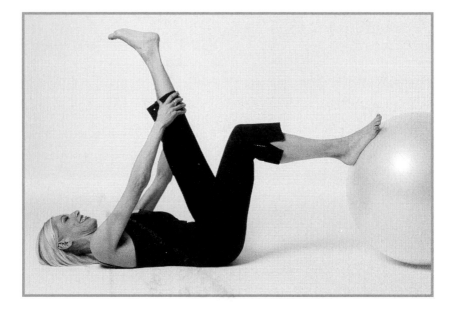

Do the right, then the left leg, and repeat, a minimum of twice on each side, holding for 30 seconds each time.

 Watchpoint: You'll know if you are doing this wrong if your bottom lifts. If this is impossible, instead of using your hands, take a towel, place it around your calf and ease the leg towards you, keeping your neck and shoulders relaxed.

Don't pull on your leg so that your bottom leaves the floor, as your pelvis will twist. You want to flex the foot without overly tensing the feet, and gently straighten that knee. It is more important to get your knee straighter than to bring the leg closer to you.

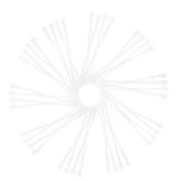

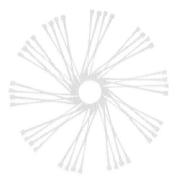

Upper Body Toning

Press-ups

Now you're ready to continue with your upper body toning and strengthening. Kneel down with your hands on the floor in front of the ball, and feet behind the ball. Carefully walk forwards until your hips are on the ball and feet off the floor. Your hands are under your shoulders – just wider than shoulder-width apart, with the palms flat and fingers pointing away from you. Keeping your head in line, gently tip your weight forwards.

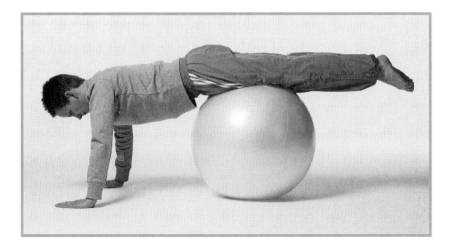

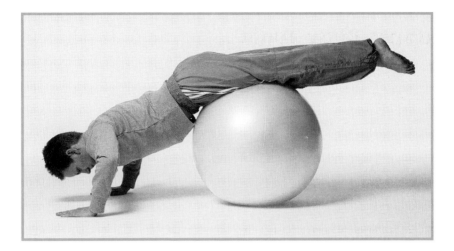

Breathe in as you bend the arms, breathe out as you straighten them, engaging your navel towards your spine.

Repeat 10 times.

 Watchpoint: The alignment of your neck and upper back is essential. Try not to seesaw and let your legs go up and down. As well as toning arms and upper back, this is essential for core stability and abdominal control.

The further over the ball you are, the less stable you are and the harder you have to work to stop your back arching.

Keep your legs together and your inner thighs gently squeezed to feel more stable.

Triceps Press

You will need a hand-weight for this one (if you haven't got one, a tin of beans or plastic bottle of water will do).

Place your right hand on the ball and kneel behind it, your left arm holding the weight. Keep your neck in line with the rest of your body.

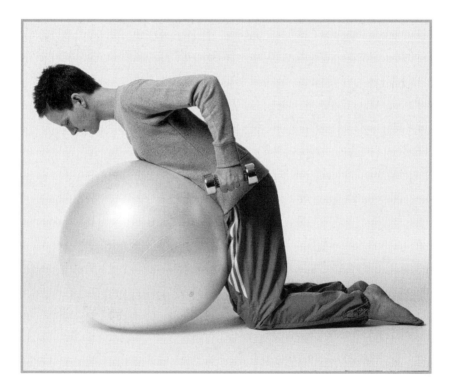

Holding the hand-weight, breathe in as you lift your left elbow up as high as you can, keeping the elbow bent at a right angle, without twisting your body. Exhale as you straighten your arm behind you. Pause. Bend your arm back again. Re-peat 10-15 times on each arm (one set). If you like you may do a second set.

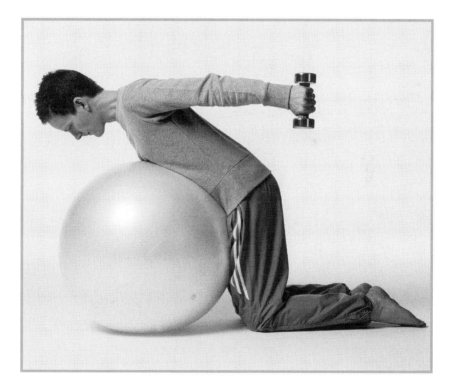

Biceps Curl

Sit on the ball with a two-kilo weight in each hand, breathe in and bend your right arm up to shoulder level. Breathe out and straighten to waist level. Try not to rock from side to side as you do this. Repeat 10 to 15 times with alternate arms. It is better to start with lighter weights if you have any doubts about the strength in your neck and shoulders.

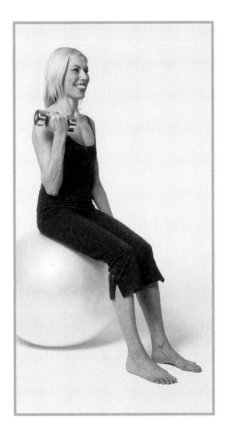

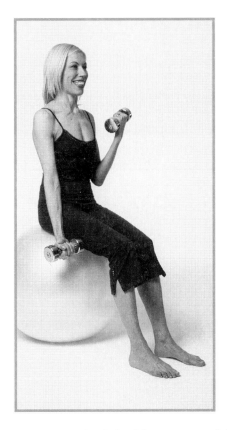

To make this sequence harder, slowly build to two sets of three exercises: 15 press-ups, 15 triceps presses on each arm, and 15 bicep curls on each arm.

 Watchpoint: At no point allow your back to arch – the focus is firstly abdominal stability and then toning the relevant muscle groups.

Shoulder Stretch

After this upper body strengthening, it is important to stretch out your shoulders. Sit in correct alignment on the ball.

Holding your arms up in front of your face, cross one over the other and clasp your hands together. Then gently push your elbows to the ceiling and feel your shoulders stretching apart. As you raise your arms, keep your shoulders down and hold this position for a count of 10. Repeat this stretch four times, alternating arms.

We are now going to do shoulder stretches with the ball in a kneeling position. For those of you who have any discomfort in your knees or lower back, I have included an exercise (Alternative Double Shoulder Stretch, page 110) where you push the ball up a wall instead.

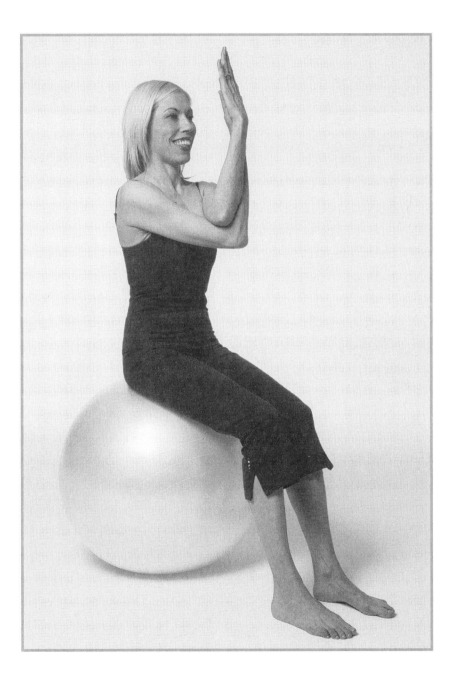

Single Shoulder Stretch

For this first shoulder stretch, you are kneeling down. Your bottom is resting on your heels. If you feel you have very tight feet and your feet are uncomfortable, you can put a towel under your feet.

Place the palm of your right hand on the centre of the ball and breathe in.

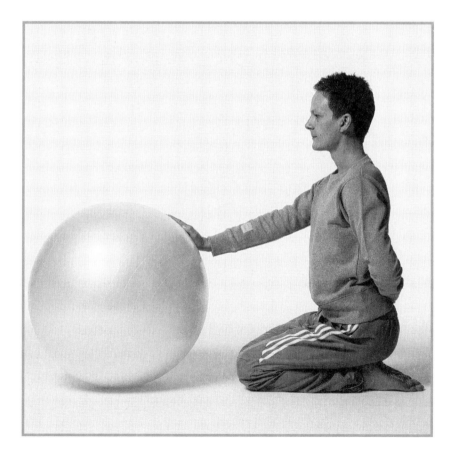

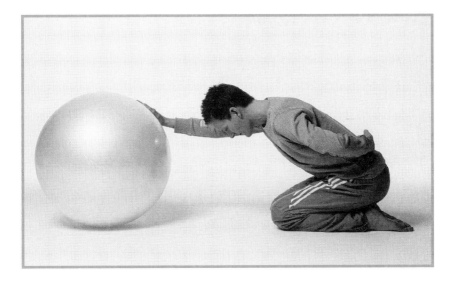

As you breathe out, push the ball as far as it will go without lifting your bottom.

Breathe in and come back to an upright position.

Do 10 repetitions on each arm.

Watchpoint: As you breathe out, feel the shoulder stretching, the shoulder blade gliding up towards your ear, then relaxing back as you breathe in. Your head and neck should just flow along the arm in a relaxed, soft movement. If your neck feels uncomfortable, you are probably in the wrong position, so adjust until your neck feels comfortable. Your elbow should not be locked at any point.

Double Shoulder Stretch

The next exercise is much more challenging. Start with the same position as the single shoulder stretch, but place both hands on the ball. Breathe in, then as you breathe out push the ball away from you and your chest towards the floor, your bottom lifting off your heels. Breathe in and come back.

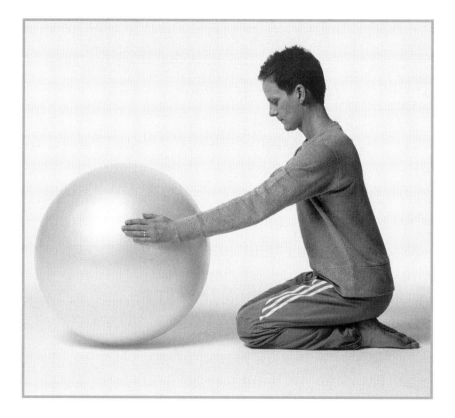

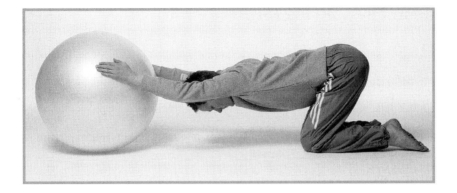

 Watchpoint: Your ears should be relaxed between your arms the whole time. Most people drop their head too low. It's just as important not to lift your head too high, so that you feel a pinching in your neck. If you feel any discomfort in your lower back, you are pushing the ball too far away.

Do not let your feet leave the ground.

Alternative Double Shoulder Stretch

This is the alternative to the above kneeling exercise, useful for anyone with either bad knees or a serious lumbar condition. It is exactly the same exercise except that you are pushing the ball up a wall.

Stand with complete Pilates postural integrity, feet hip-width apart, stomach in, tail-bone dropped, head and neck in line, arms raised with your ears between your arms, elbows released. Breathe in.

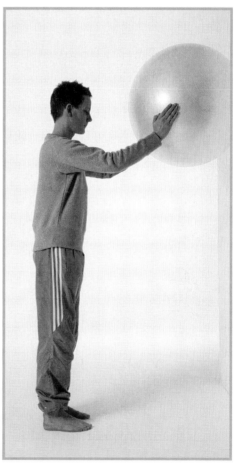

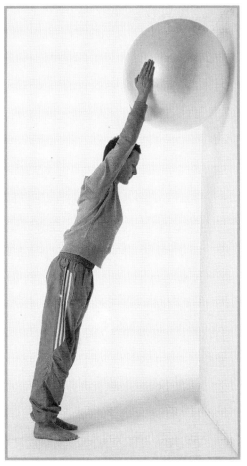

As you breathe out, push the ball up the wall. Make sure your abdominals are engaged so there is no arching in your lower back.

Repeat 10 times.

Watchpoint: If you are too far away from the wall your heels will come off the ground and your back will arch. If you are too close you will not feel the stretch.

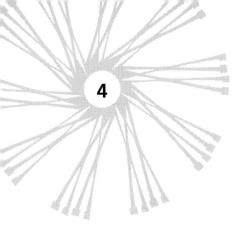

4

Pilates for Pregnancy

Exercising during Pregnancy

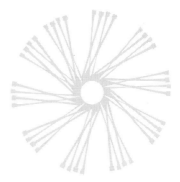

The pregnancy exercises that I've included in this book are the ones that my clients have been doing for several years on a day-to-day basis. Some of my clients have been through four successful pregnancies with me. On an average week the studio can have anywhere between 10 and 15 clients who are expecting a baby. And after a certain period they all come back, usually between three and six months after the birth, to get their bodies back in shape.

The exercises shown in this book are only the sequence of exercises we do using the ball. In the studio we do a lot of other equipment-based work and mat work that is not included in this book.

I cannot stress how important it is that each pregnancy is different. Whether it is your first or your fourth or more, you must always listen to what your body is telling you. If you are tired at any point, rest. If you are hungry, eat. As I say to all my pregnant clients, the most important thing is a healthy mother and baby.

Exercises that may be perfectly fine one day may feel uncomfortable the next. This depends a lot on the way the baby is lying. Obviously, as the pregnancy develops you must listen to your body and, if any exercise makes you feel uncomfortable, you must stop. If you get any discomfort, particularly around the base of your abdominals, around your pubic bone or your pelvic floor muscles, that is an indication that you need to stop exercising.

It is important only to exercise after first checking with your doctor and any other healthcare professionals you may be seeing during your pregnancy. I feel it is necessary also to stress that if it is your first baby then you are much less aware of your body – any discomfort, nausea, any of the changes that the body naturally undergoes during pregnancy. In my studio – and doctors will also advise this – it is recommended that for up to the first three months you should not undertake a new exercise programme. The risk of miscarriage is always higher during the first three months of pregnancy. Obviously, if your healthcare professional suggests that you do something, for instance swimming, that is a different issue. In my studio the clients who are pregnant always have priority of both my and my staff's attention. If you have any doubts at all about any of the exercises, I would much prefer you didn't do them.

Particularly in modern society for women of this century, pregnancy realistically is a very small part of your life. It is important not to pressurize yourself to keep fit, to overexercise, to worry about the shape of your body. Yes, you are having a baby. This means you are going to get larger. It is totally feasible to regain your body shape after pregnancy without worrying unduly about media images of pregnancy. Whenever any of my clients says, 'I'm fat' – I say, 'You are not fat, you are pregnant.' I will restate that a healthy mother and baby is what we all desire.

After the birth I always insist that my clients do not exercise until they have had their six-week check-up. This does not mean that if your healthcare professionals give you (which they normally do) pelvic floor exercises under their personal direction that you shouldn't do these. What I am saying is, until you have had your six-week check-up your body is still at a vulnerable point and you need to take care of yourself. This also involves anything like heavy lifting, because your body is still under stress from the birth.

It can be up to the first year after the birth of a baby that the relaxin hormones are still in your body. So it is important to tailor your exercise programme with this in mind. You may feel fine now, but you may want to think about how your body may feel in 10 years if you overstress it when it is still vulnerable to the after-effects of childbirth. I cannot stress too strongly that the media images of women getting their bodies back immediately after birth are *not* the norm. Some of my clients return to their natural shape within three months, some take six to eight months. This depends on the individual concerned. Also, the older you are the harder it is for the body to bounce back.

It is also quite important to remember that it is very difficult to get back to what you might think of as your pre-pregnancy weight if you are breastfeeding. As we know, nursing is an essential part of a child's development. Most of my clients who breastfeed don't actually return to their natural weight until slightly after those who, for whatever reason, haven't breastfed their babies. If you are nursing, obviously you have you eat more because you are feeding yourself *and* the baby.

Every pregnancy is different, every birth is different, and every body is different, so it is important not to have unreal images of what you expect your body to look like before or after the birth. The main thing I want to stress is that you should be able to enjoy this phase of your life. You have made a positive choice to have a baby and it should be a joyous experience.

Pilates and Pregnancy

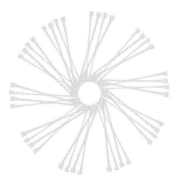

**Jane Ireland MCSP SRP,
Chartered Physiotherapist**

For a mother, the birth of a child is a truly miraculous event. What I find even more remarkable are the physiological changes the body goes through from conception to birth, and how the mother's body recovers afterwards.

Pregnancy is not a disease or an illness, it is a condition which should be managed for the sake of the baby's development and the mother's well-being. A mother who is suffering from low back pain, pelvic instability, upper back or arm pain will not enjoy looking after her newborn baby.

Pregnancy puts great physical demands on the mother's body. Effective Pilates during and after pregnancy helps to support the body physically during pregnancy, and vitally helps the physical recovery afterwards.

From the early days of pregnancy, a hormone called *relaxin* is released into the body to help with the 'softening' of the ligaments. This enables the mother's body to 'grow' comfortably to accommodate the increasingly large foetus. With increasing laxity in the body ligaments, the joints are more vulnerable to the normal stresses and strains of everyday life. The mother's necessary increase in weight is also loading up her frame.

The human muscle system is trainable – that is, we can make it work to our advantage to help give stability and strength to a mother's body. However, it must be recognized that *not all exercise is beneficial.*

Pilates works on all muscle groups in a biomechanically correct way, so preventing overworking of some and underworking of other muscle groups, which can lead to an imbalanced muscle system and one which is prone to injury.

The basis of all Pilates is core stability (co-contracting of the pelvic floor and deep abdominal muscles). These muscles help control the pelvis and give support to the spine. Core stability exercises do not mean sit-ups; it is potentially dangerous to do sit-ups while pregnant. Lesley makes you work the core muscles in various challenging ways without putting you or your baby at risk.

Pregnancy often causes the mother's posture to change to more of a swaying-forward, slouched-shoulders presentation. This again makes you more vulnerable to pain and injury. Posture is constantly worked on at the Body Maintenance studio, both with strength work, flexibility and body awareness.

Immediately after the birth of your child, gentle pelvic floor exercises should be started, but for any other exercise you should wait a minimum of six weeks. Pilates post-pregnancy will help to get your pelvic floor and abdominal control back; it will help to stabilize your spine, strengthen your upper body to help with the continual lifting of the baby, and – probably most noticeably of all – it will help you to get your body shape back!

I started doing Pilates at Body Maintenance just before my second pregnancy. I continued throughout the pregnancy, working on, among other things, core muscles, spinal strength and flexibility, leg strength and flexibility, arm strength and postural exercises. After my son was born I started again, initially with just a few exercises at home concentrating on the pelvic floor, then, as time allowed, in the studio. Lesley works you hard, and the work is extremely effective. Each individual programme is designed to each woman's particular needs. The rewards are plenty: my body shape has come back – something I never thought would happen, having had two rather large baby boys! I feel stronger than I have in a long time, my posture is better, and I feel better in myself. Lesley – thank you.

First Movements

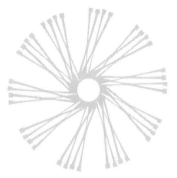

Bouncing on the Ball

For this first exercise you are seated on the ball, your tailbone heavy and both feet evenly placed on the floor, hip-width apart. You are in contact from your centre directly down through your feet into the floor. You are going to channel your energies from your centre out through the crown of your head. Your shoulders and arms are relaxed. Your tailbone will relax and your abdominals will naturally drop back towards your spine.

Rather than pulling your tummy in, imagine the baby dropping back into your spine. Try to think of your head sitting naturally on top of your shoulders, neither pushing it forward nor pulling it back.

Gently bounce on the ball for anywhere up to 3 minutes.

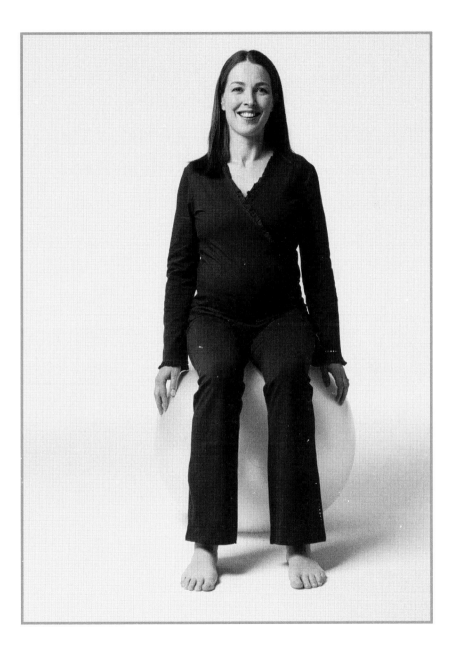

Single Shoulder Stretches

These relax your shoulders and neck.

Sit comfortably on the ball with your arms relaxed at your sides. Breathe in and slowly squeeze your right shoulder up to your right ear. Breathe out and relax your shoulder down. Repeat with the other shoulder. Do this to a count of four up, four down. Don't move your head.

Repeat 10 times, alternating shoulders.

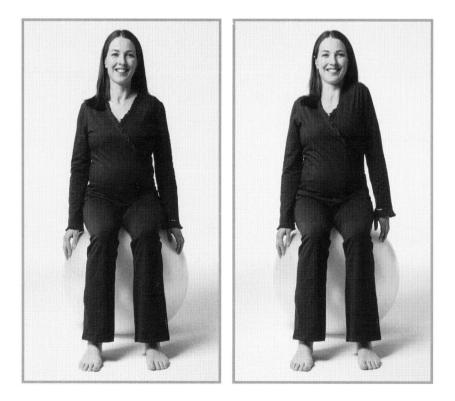

Double Shoulder Stretches

Sitting as above, squeeze both shoulders up to your ears. Make sure your hands are dangling loosely by your sides. Repeat 10 times.

 Watchpoint: It is important not to lock your elbows or stick your neck forward.

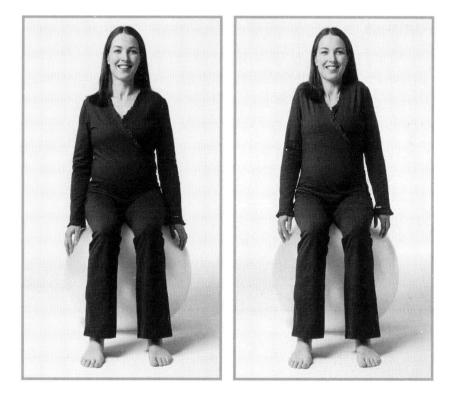

Shoulder Circles

Assume the same position as above. Place your hands on your shoulders and very gently circle both arms forward.

Repeat 10 times.

Circle your arms backwards, again repeating 10 times.

If this feels uncomfortable, circle your shoulders with your arms at your sides.

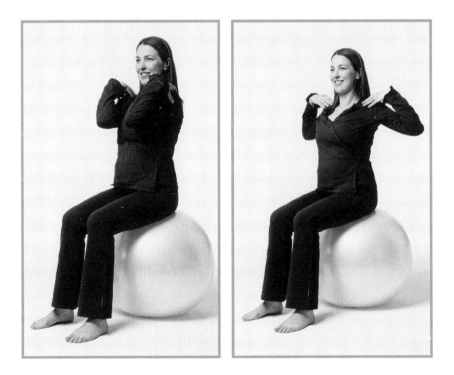

Pelvic Floor

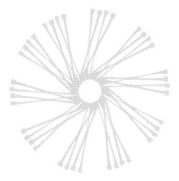

The reason you're working your pelvic floor muscles is that you want to keep the baby from dropping for as long as possible. You also need strong pelvic floor muscles to take the pressure off your bladder and bowel, which can cause discomfort as the baby develops and gets heavier. My clients do very minimal exercises lying on their backs after the first 14 weeks of pregnancy. There is only one included in this programme, which my clients do right up to full-term.

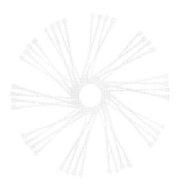

Pelvic Floor Exercise 1

This is like a pelvic tilt, but rather than lying down you sit on the ball, hands on your hips. Breathe in and then, very gently as you breathe out, tip your pelvis under. Do not pull your stomach in, but imagine the baby dropping in towards your spine.

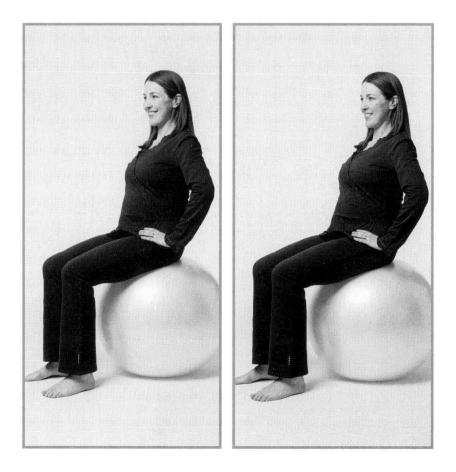

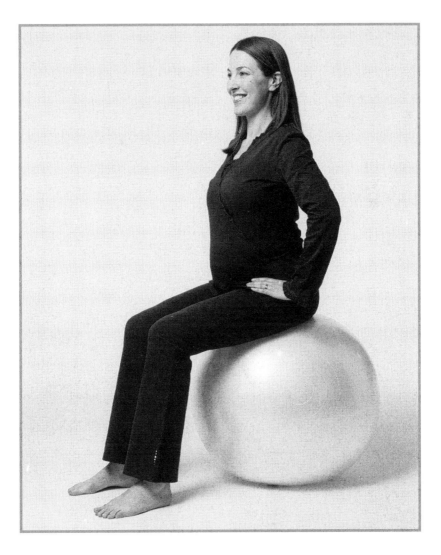

Breathe in and arch the other way. Breathe out. Let the ball roll under you.

Repeat about 10 times.

Pelvic Floor Exercise 2

People often find these next two exercises quite difficult to start with. What you're trying to do is tighten the muscles around your pubic bone, the base of your abdominals.

Seated on the ball as in the previous exercise, breathe in, take your arms above your head, breathe out and curl gently back. Allow the baby to drop into your spine and you will feel a tightening round the base of your pubic bone. Breathe in and sit up without arching your back. Breathe in, with your arms up. Breathe out, drop back over the ball, feel the baby drop and feel a tightening round your pubic bone.

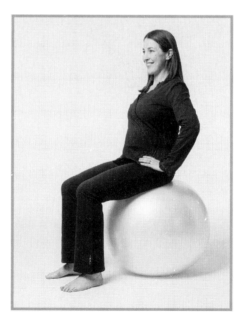

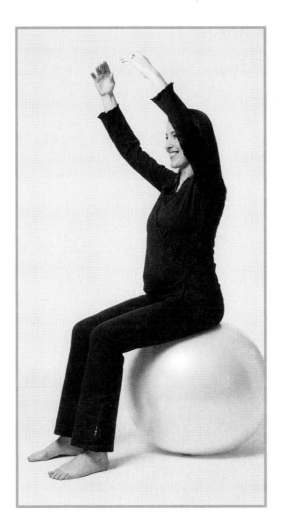

Do approximately 10 repetitions.

It can be helpful to think of gently tightening your inner thighs as you breathe out, as this will connect with your pelvic floor muscles.

Pelvic Floor Exercise 3

This exercise is very similar to the last one. Put your left hand around your waist. Breathe in, breathe out, think of the baby dropping back in towards your spine and raise your right arm.

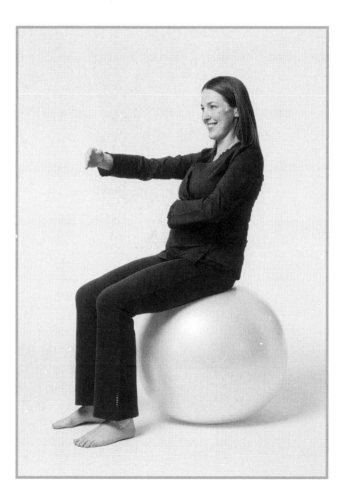

You will feel the muscles round your waist contracting as you lower your right arm, also the muscles round the pubic bone, the pelvic floor muscles. Breathe in and curl up.

Do 10 repetitions with alternating arms.

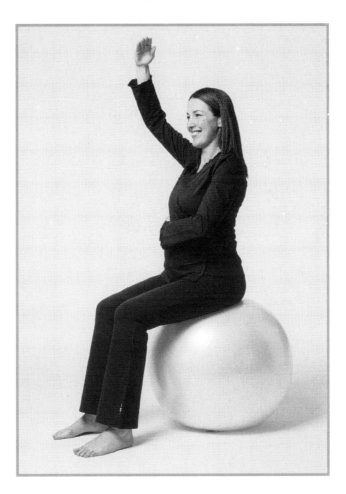

Pelvic Floor Strengthening

The next exercise is done on your hands and knees. Have the ball supported by a wall. Kneel in a comfortable position so your hands are supported by the ball. Keep your head and neck in line, and your back flat like a table-top. Your knees should be under your hips. Take a small towel between your thighs.

Breathe in, and as you breathe out squeeze the towel between your inner thighs. You will feel the base of your stomach contracting around your pelvic floor muscles. Do not allow your back to arch.

Repeat about 10 times.

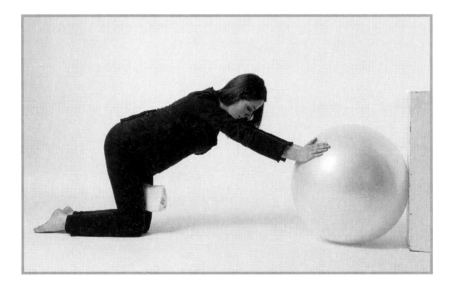

Watchpoint: It is impossible to pull your stomach in when you are pregnant. Don't think stomach – think of the deep pelvic floor muscles between the point of your anus and the point of your pubic bone.

If you feel any discomfort in your knees, place a towel beneath them. Make sure you are securely positioned on the ball and that you feel stable before you start.

This is an exercise you could quite easily do a second set of later in your programme or at a completely different time during the day.

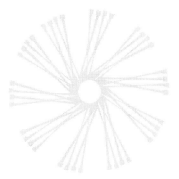

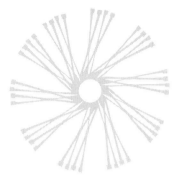

Back and Thighs

Hip Rolls

This is a mobilization exercise for your spine, to keep it supple.

Lie on your back with your feet on the ball, feet and legs together and tail-bone on the floor. Your ankles and knees should be in line with your hips, and your feet relaxed.

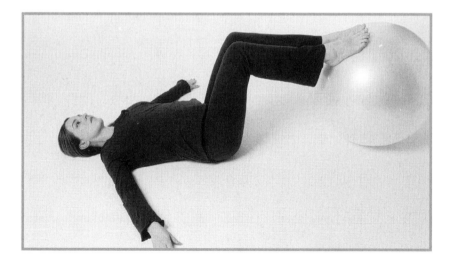

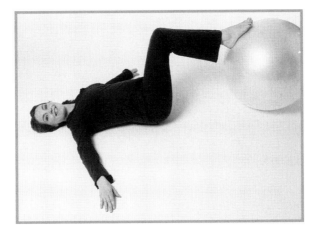

Breathe in and, as you breathe out, let your legs go one way but keep your head in the centre. Breathe in and bring your legs back to centre. Repeat in the opposite direction. At no point move your head, nor let your shoulder blades come off the mat. Keep it a small, controlled movement. Start by doing 10 in total – that is, 5 to each side.

Watchpoint: Do not let the ball take you any further than your shoulders can control the movement. I must stress that this is a very small movement. The most important part of this exercise is that at no point should either shoulder blade leave the mat. Your knees should stay together as you move from side to side – this way one leg won't get longer than the other. It is very natural as you turn from side to side to take your knees further than your ankles.

Cat Stretch

This exercise will release your lower back and stretch out your shoulders.

Support the ball against a wall. Kneel as far away as you can while still resting your palms on the ball. Keep your weight distributed evenly through to your knees. Keep your hips over your knees.

Breathe in and, as you breathe out, curl your chin into your chest and stretch out your lower back.

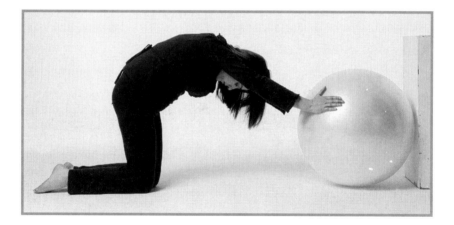

As you breathe in, press your chest down, your bottom up and gently lengthen your neck.

This counts as one repetition. Repeat 10 times.

As you open your spine, this gets the blood flowing and will counteract the effects of gravity, altering your spinal integrity as the baby develops – otherwise your lower back can become over-extended, which can lead to backache and, in some cases, sciatica.

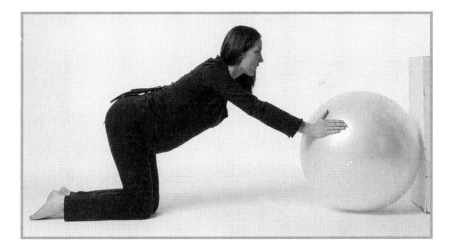

 Watchpoint: If you feel your neck crunching or your vocal cords contracting, you've taken your head too far back. There should be no discomfort in your neck.

Make sure your feet stay on the floor.

Inside Thigh Exercise 1

You do this one lying on your side, preferably with your back supported by a wall, and with the arm that's on the floor either supporting your head or completely flat. If you choose to keep your arm flat, it may feel more comfortable to put a towel between your arm and ear. Your other hand should be in front of you. Your top leg should be forward, in front of your body, with your foot on the ball. The underneath leg (the one that is working) needs to be slightly forward, with your foot gently flexed. Don't lock your knee, but pull up the muscles so that your leg is straight. If your legs are not straight, you'll be working your ankle and your foot much more than your inside thigh.

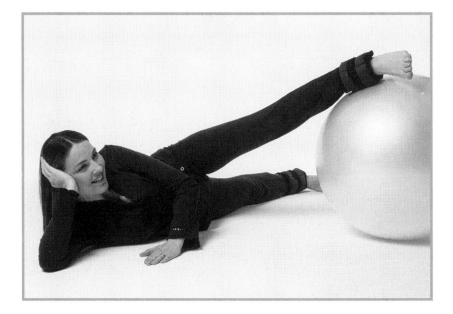

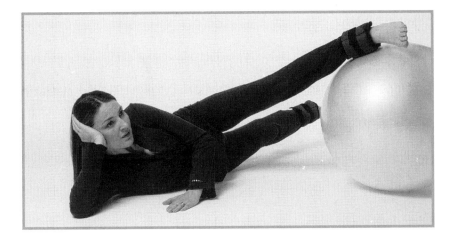

Lie on your left side and breathe in. As you breathe out, lift your left leg and hold. As you lift and breathe out, feel your waist toning as well as your inner thigh. The energy is through your heel, working your inner thigh.

Do 10 with your left leg, then turn onto your right side and do 10 with your right leg.

Watchpoint: It is important for this exercise, particularly after the fifth month of pregnancy, that you lie with your back against a wall so that both hips are supported by it and there is no strain in your lumbar spine. It will probably be more comfortable for you with your head on your arm.

Make sure your hips are in line, 'stacked' one on top of the other.

Inside Thigh Lift 2

Lie on your left side, as in the above exercise. Lift your left leg, bend your knee gently and 'squeeze' to straighten your leg. Keep your foot gently flexed and your knee unlocked. You may want to place a small towel between your arm and your ear for comfort.

Repeat 10 times, keeping your leg in the air the whole time as you bend it.

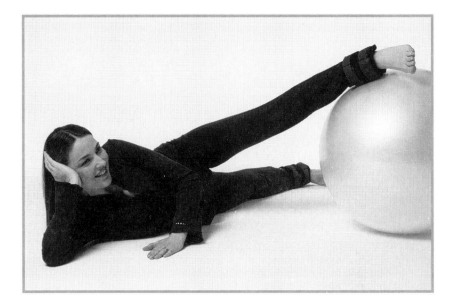

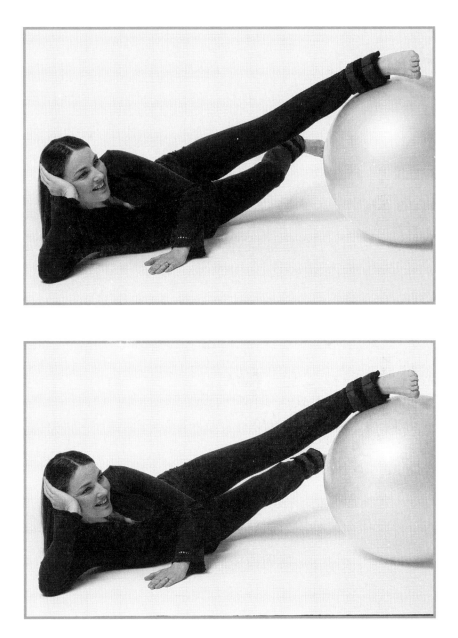

Upper Body

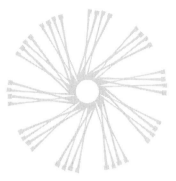

Press-ups

Now you're ready to continue with your upper body toning and strengthening. Kneel down with your hands on the floor in front of the ball, your feet behind the ball.

Carefully walk forwards until your hips are on the ball and your feet are off the floor. Only go as far over the ball as feels comfortable. Your hands are under your shoulders – just wider than shoulder-width apart, with the palms flat and fingers pointing away from you. Keeping your head in line, gently tip your weight forwards.

Breathe in as you bend your arms, breathe out as you straighten them, keeping your back stable.

Repeat 10 times.

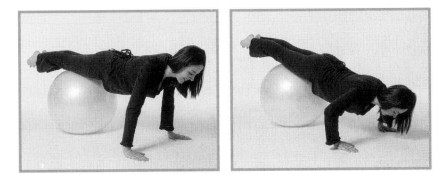

Watchpoint: The further over the ball you are, the less stable you are and the harder you have to work. Keep your legs together and your inside thighs gently squeezed to feel more stable. It's very important not to arch your back.

The alignment of your neck and upper back is essential. Try not to seesaw or let your legs go up and down. As well as toning arms and upper back, this is essential for core stability.

This is an exercise you must use your judgement on. Some of my clients carry on doing this up until quite late stages of pregnancy, some do not. Slightly later on in the programme you will see an alternative press-up against a wall. If you have any discomfort around where the baby is lying, do the Alternative Press-ups (page 154).

Triceps Press

Make sure the ball is secured by a wall. Place your left hand on the ball and kneel behind it, keeping your right arm straight to the ground. Keep your neck in line with the rest of your body. Holding a hand weight (a tin of beans or bottle of water will do), inhale and lift your right elbow up as high as you can, keeping your elbow bent at a right angle, without twisting your body. Exhale as you straighten your arm behind you. Pause. Bend your arm back again. Hold the ball and lean as far over the ball as you feel secure.

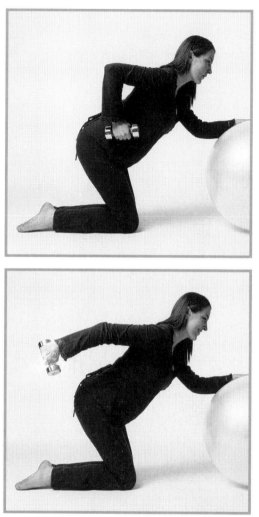

Repeat 10-15 times on each arm (this is one 'set'). You may do a second set.

Watchpoint: At no point allow your back to arch.

Biceps Curl

Sit on the ball with a 2-kilo weight in each hand. Breathe in and bend your arm up to shoulder level. Breathe out and straighten to waist level. Try not to rock as you do this. Repeat 10 to 15 times with alternate arms.

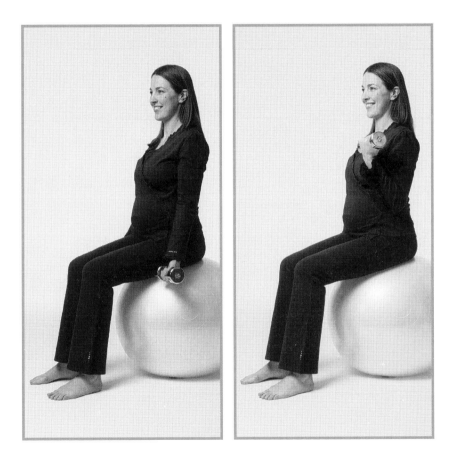

Legs and Bottom

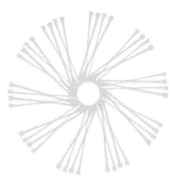

Standing Calf Stretch

Stand up straight, holding the ball in your hands and positioned against a wall. Take a step forward with your left leg and, leaning against the ball, bend your knee slightly and feel the stretch down through your right leg. Keep your right heel down. Do not bounce. Hold for 30 seconds. Repeat 4 times, alternating legs.

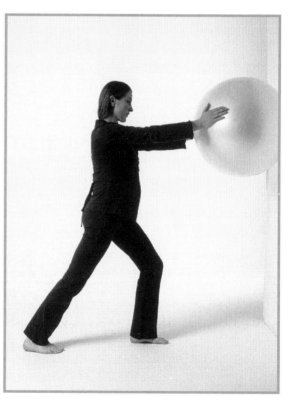

Quadriceps Stretch

Kneel down on your right leg, keeping your back straight, and rest your hands on the ball, which should be supported against a solid surface. Then extend your left leg straight, making sure that your heel is always in front of your knee. Gently relax the baby into your spine and lean back slightly, making sure you don't arch your back. Hold for 30 seconds.

Repeat twice for each leg.

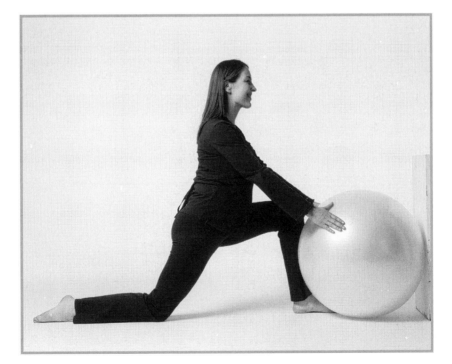

Seated Buttock Stretch

This is one of only two exercises not on the ball, as using the ball would be too unstable.

Seated on a chair, starting with both feet on the ground, raise and cross your right ankle over your left knee. Breathe in, then very gently breathe out and lean forward. Try to lean over your bent (right) knee and you will feel a stretch in the back of your hip and buttock. Keep your head, neck and shoulders relaxed. Hold for 20 seconds.

Gently press your right knee down, without either pulling on your ankle and foot or twisting your pelvis. If this feels uncomfortable, you can always put your left foot on a telephone directory to lift it slightly higher. Repeat 4 times on each leg, alternating legs.

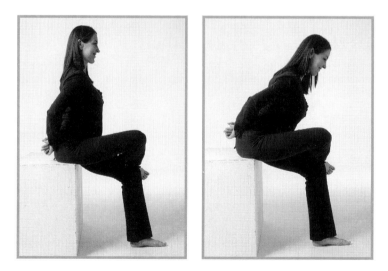

Watchpoint: It is absolutely vital to stretch out the back of the hip muscles when you are pregnant, due to the fact that gravity is constantly creating an over-arched lumbar spine, which can cause lumbar and back problems and sciatica. Basically, my pregnant clients don't get sciatica because we do a huge amount of mobilization and strengthening to avoid a strain in the lumbar spine. This can be caused by the change in posture, the problems with gravity as the body changes and the weight of the baby constantly tipping you forward.

Buttock-Toning

Many of my clients do the earlier buttock-toning exercises over the ball (pages 89, 90 and 91) up to the point where they no longer feel comfortable on the ball. Again, you can use your judgement during your earlier stages of pregnancy.

Stronger Stretches

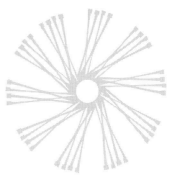

Standing Hamstring Stretch

This exercise will stretch the back of your legs. You must make sure that whatever you are using to support your leg is a very stable surface. The height of the box or whatever you use is relevant to how tight your legs are. This varies from person to person. And as you get bigger, you may need to change the height, possibly taking it lower.

Place your right foot, gently flexed, on a stable surface and extend your leg. Keep your left leg slightly bent and your neck and shoulders relaxed. Hips are level. Slide your hands down towards your right foot. You should feel the stretch in the muscle between your knee and the hip. Hold for 20 seconds.

Repeat 4 times, alternating legs.

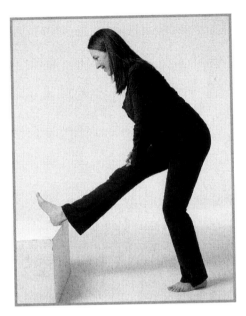

 Watchpoint: Keep the leg you are standing on slightly bent.

It is really important when you are pregnant that you don't do developmental stretching, because the ligaments and the tendons soften to allow for the birth of the baby. A lot of people get confused and think that they are actually more flexible. This is not true. If you over-stretch a tendon or ligament during pregnancy, it will remain overstretched after the birth. The female body is perfectly designed for everything to return to normal after giving birth, but obviously not if you have overstretched.

Alternative Press-ups

Have the ball supported by a wall, with your palms as wide as possible on the ball slightly below shoulder level. Breathe in as you bend your elbows and come towards the ball, breathe out as you straighten.

Repeat about 10 times – but as this is less demanding than press-ups over the ball, do an extra set when you feel comfortable with the exercise.

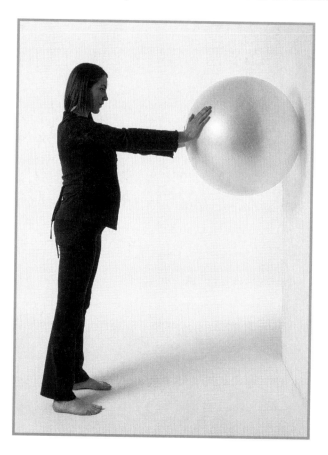

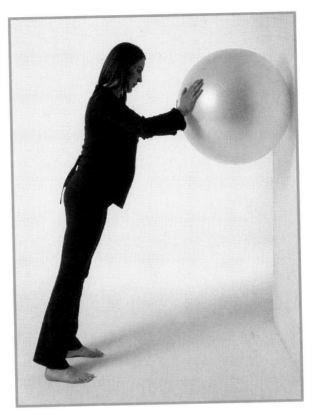

 Watchpoint: Keep your neck and shoulders in line.

Do not arch your lower back.

You will know if you are too far away from the ball, as your heels will leave the ground.

Single Shoulder Stretch

For this first shoulder stretch, you are kneeling down. Your bottom is resting on your heels. If you feel you have very tight feet and/or your feet are uncomfortable, you can put a towel under them.

Place the palm of your left hand on the centre of the ball. As you breathe out, push the ball as far as it will go without lifting your bottom. Breathe in and come back to an upright position. As you breathe out feel your shoulder stretching, the shoulder blade gliding up towards your ear, then relaxing back as you breathe in.

Let your head and neck just flow along your arm in a relaxed, soft movement. If your neck feels uncomfortable you are probably in the wrong position, so adjust it until your neck feels comfortable. Your elbow should not be locked at any point.

Do 10 repetitions on each arm.

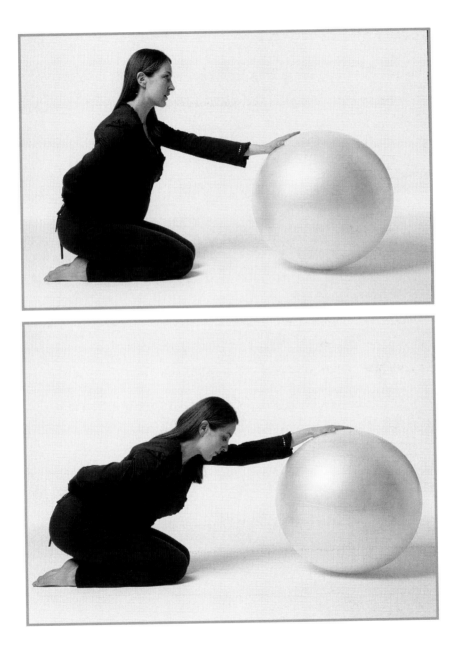

Double Shoulder Stretch

This next exercise is much more challenging. Start in the same position as for the single shoulder stretch, but place both hands on the sides of the ball. Breathe in, then as you breathe out push the ball away from you, pushing your chest to the floor as your bottom comes off your heels. Breathe in and come back.

Watchpoint: Keep your ears relaxed between your arms the whole time. Most people drop their head too low. It's just as important not to lift your head too high so you feel a pinching in your neck.

Do not let your feet leave the ground.

This is an upper body stretch, so if you feel any discomfort in your lower back, you are working incorrectly and pushing the ball too far away.

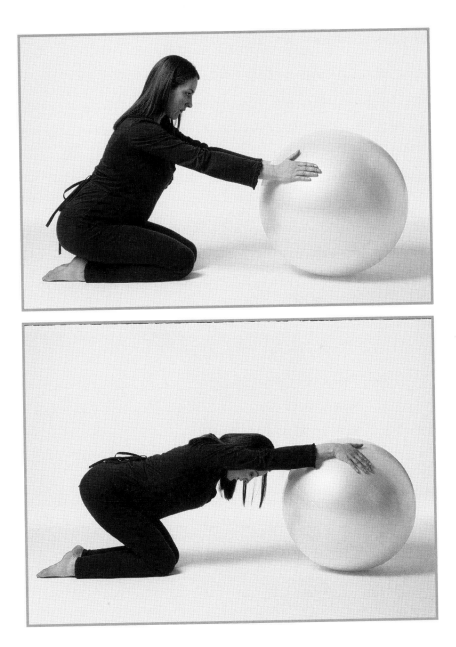

Alternative Ball Stretch

This is the alternative to the above kneeling exercise, useful for anyone with either bad knees or a serious lumbar condition. It is exactly the same exercise except that you push the ball up a wall. Many of my pregnant clients replace the kneeling shoulder stretch with this standing wall stretch as their pregnancy develops.

Stand with complete Pilates postural integrity, feet hip-width apart, tailbone dropped, head and neck in line, ears between your raised arms, elbows released.

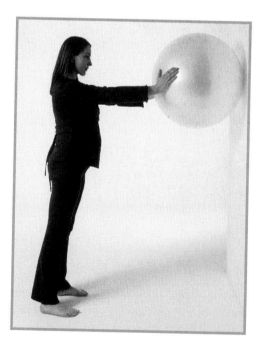

Breathe in and, as you breathe out, push the ball up the wall. Do not lock your elbows, do not arch your back. Make sure the ball is against a secure surface.

Repeat 10 times.

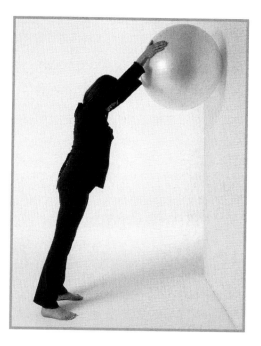

 Watchpoint: If you are too far away from the wall your heels will come off the ground and your back will arch. If you are too close you will not get any stretch.

One Mother's Story: Julia Daly

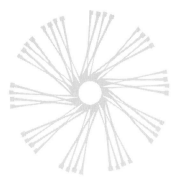

Julia Daly started taking Lesley's classes to help with her recurring lower back pain, then discovered how it helped her through her second pregnancy:

'I started seeing Lesley about seven months after the birth of my first son, Louis. My lower back would go into spasms and I wouldn't be able to move for three, sometimes five days. I'd have to take a lot of painkillers and be carried in to see an osteopath. I was worried about the pain getting worse with a child in tow. Although I was sceptical that Pilates could help with such chronic pain, I have not had to visit the osteopath once since I started my sessions, twice a week, in 1999.

'When I got pregnant again Lesley devised a suitable programme for me. We concentrated on the pelvic floor and some very gentle stomach exercises. These were done by lifting the stomach towards the spine, flattening it rather than contracting the stomach muscles. About 13 weeks into my pregnancy Lesley stopped me from doing any exercises on my back because the weight of the baby would put pressure on major veins. I continued with all the arm and leg exercises, and some modified waist exercises, using the Physio Ball. Lesley tailored the programme to my body type as well: because I have long legs and a relatively short back, she would make sure I wouldn't lift my legs too high, for example. She always erred on the side of caution and made sure I didn't overextend myself. As the sessions were strengthening but nonetheless fairly gentle, I was showing up regularly right up until I started getting contractions. Lesley sent me home even though I was prepared to stay and finish the class! Two days later I gave birth to my second son, Freddie. I'm now pregnant again and see no reason not do the same this time round as well.

'My second pregnancy was much easier because of Pilates. As it's a lengthening programme, I felt that I had room in my body for my baby. Some pregnant women can't eat full meals towards the end of their pregnancy, but I never felt like my body was being overtaken by this child. By strengthening my spine and maintaining my posture through Pilates I was able to resist another common problem of the back arching inwards, which also causes terrible back pains.

'During my first pregnancy I often felt I was tuned in to eight radio stations at once, with my mind constantly worrying about so many things at the same time. Attending two 90-minute classes a week during my second pregnancy really helped me take my mind off everything else and focus on just one thing, because the exercises require so much concentration, which was also very relaxing. I would come into each session after I'd been rushing around and I would leave feeling very at peace with myself.

'Although I don't work up a sweat as I would in an aerobics class, I always feel I've worked out after Pilates. As a low-impact strengthening programme it definitely helped when it came to labour, as I felt I could ride the exhaustion out more easily. If you stop breastfeeding quite soon then you can go back to exercising on a more rigorous basis, but I did it gradually, and six months after Freddie was born I was completely back to normal. Despite carrying two heavy boys all the time, my back has never felt stronger. I don't have the aches and pains of my other friends who have children.

'Many pregnant women don't get their waistline back, but with Pilates my waist is better than it has ever been. I really like the body shape Pilates has given me. It has broadened my shoulder line, nipped in my waist and really lengthened me. Lesley's arm exercises have also prevented my bust from travelling south! I'm toned but it doesn't look "worked", and that's all due to the Pilates. People think I've lost weight, even though I haven't. It's like I've redistributed the weight in a nicer fashion.'

15-Minute Pilates

Body maintenance to make you longer, leaner and stronger

Lesley Ackland

Many fitness enthusiasts have found that some exercise techniques can lead to over-developed muscles, making their bodies less streamlined and elegant. Pilates is different.

Traditionally popular with ballet dancers and models, it gives you a longer, leaner physique, better posture, a strong back and more mobility. It is soft exercise that combines low-impact but high energy movements with realignment of posture.

Lesley Ackland has developed a 'body maintenance' programme that helps a wide range of problems, including back pain, scoliosis, RSI, arthritis, pregnancy and stress problems. The cleverly-devised 15-minute-a-day programme can be tailored to suit your own needs and will make a world of difference to your looks and your health.

Pilates Over 50

Longer, Leaner, Stronger, Younger

Lesley Ackland

Lesley Ackland, a fantastic advertisement for the power of Pilates, looks 20 years younger thanks to her age-defying Pilates body maintenance system. In Pilates Over 50, she shares her fitness and nutrition secrets so anyone can look and feel years younger.

Pilates is the perfect exercise regime for the over 50s. The simple, low-impact exercises in Lesley's exercise programme will make you longer, leaner and stronger for life, bringing you fantastic long-term health benefits.

- Maintain flexible pain-free joints and a strong back
- Improve bone density and prevent osteoporosis
- Alleviate arthritis and other age-related problems
- Improve posture
- Tone and lengthen muscles so clothes look great
- Move with suppleness and grace to make you look even younger

With nutritional advice as well as the exercises Lesley's clients have used to alleviate age-related problems, this comprehensive guide will keep you looking and feeling young for life.

10-Step Pilates

Reshape your body and transform your life

Leslie Ackland

Now you can dramatically transform your looks and your health by design-ing your own Pilates exercise programme, using 10 short regimes, to suit your needs.

10-Step Pilates encourages you to work on your body and mind through the day:

- Your body: for a toned stomach, slim long legs and a strong back
- Your moods: wake up and energize or wind down and refresh
- Your environment: exercises for home and the workplace

Make
www.thorsonselement.com
your online sanctuary

Get online information, inspiration and
guidance to help you on the path to physical
and spiritual well-being. Drawing on the integrity
and vision of our authors and titles, and with
health advice, articles, astrology, tarot, a
meditation zone, author interviews and events
listings, www.thorsonselement.com is a great
alternative to help create space and peace
in our lives.

So if you've always wondered about practising
yoga, following an allergy-free diet, using the
tarot or getting a life coach, we can point you
in the right direction.

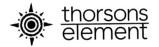

www.thorsonselement.com